# END YOUR
# MENOPAUSE
# MISERY

# END YOUR MENOPAUSE MISERY

## *the* 10-DAY Self-Care Plan

STEPHANIE BENDER

*&*

TREACY COLBERT

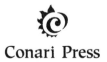

Conari Press

First published in 2013 by Conari Press
Red Wheel/Weiser, LLC
With offices at:
665 Third Street, Suite 400
San Francisco, CA 94107
*www.redwheelweiser.com*

ISBN: 978-1-57324-585-2

Library of Congress Cataloging-in-Publication Data available upon request

Cover design by Nita Ybarra
Interior by Jane Hagaman

Printed in the United States of America
MAL

10  9  8  7  6  5  4  3  2  1

The paper used in this publication meets the minimum requirements of
the American National Standard for Information Sciences—Permanence
of Paper for Printed Library Materials Z39.48-1992 (R1997).

*This book is dedicated to my sons, Billy and Tim,*
*who traveled with me through this sometimes*
*challenging part of my life's journey.*
*You never faltered in your love and encouragement of me.*
*Thank you for always being there.*

*To my grandchildren,*
*Ethan, Cade, and Kendall,*
*whose smiles and energy fueled me*
*and kept me moving forward.*

*And to my friend,*
*who made me laugh when laughter seemed impossible*
*and who brought new spontaneity to my life.*

*Each of you has played a very big part*
*in the heart and soul poured into creating this book.*

*—SB*

*"You can't turn back the clock, but you can wind it up again."*
—*Bonnie Prudden*

# CONTENTS

# FOREWORD

As a family physician, I find that a comprehensive, holistic, and personalized approach to menopause provides the best outcome for my patients. I see many women who are uncertain about how to cope with sleeplessness, depression, low libido, difficulty concentrating, hot flashes, and other signs of hormone imbalance. They worry that menopause marks the beginning of a decline. They want answers but frequently feel overwhelmed about where to begin. *End Your Menopause Misery: The 10-Day Self-Care Plan* by Stephanie Bender and Treacy Colbert fills a great need with a step-by-step plan to help you sort out what's best for you. At the end of ten days, you'll feel like you've gained a significant measure of control over your health and well-being.

Millions of women suffer daily from uncomfortable and bewildering hormonal changes associated with perimenopause and menopause, but they don't have to. Recognizing and proactively managing these symptoms become much simpler and more straightforward with *End Your Menopause Misery*. This concise guide will help you improve your health, quality of life, and relationships.

The powerful motto "one day at a time" applies to this book. Each chapter is devoted to one day, offering specific tips and strategies aimed at easing a particular menopause symptom. Clear and uncomplicated, the plan tells you what to eat, what to avoid, how to find new ways to enjoy being active, and how to think about intimacy with a renewed outlook. The discussion covers everything from restoring sound sleep to lifting your mood, increasing your heart and bone strength, and you'll find flexible recommendations that let you adapt the approach to suit your lifestyle and preferences.

*End Your Menopause Misery* also unpacks the issue of hormone replacement therapy (HRT), demystifying the subject and explaining it succinctly. After reading this book, women who choose to explore HRT with their health care provider can begin the conversation with a solid under-standing and with confidence that their decision will be well thought out and right for them.

*End Your Menopause Misery* reassures women that they can not only manage their menopause symptoms, but they can also rediscover their happier, sexier selves. I will be pleased to advise my patients to read this valuable guide to a healthy and happy stage of life.

*Enjoy,*
*Fred Grover Jr., MD*

# ACKNOWLEDGMENTS

I want to thank all the people who offered their encouragement, time, and energy to make this book possible: Treacy Colbert; Barbara Moulton; Caroline Pincus; and Fred Grover Jr., MD. Also Terri Pobanz; Rosalie Stofflet; John DeGraff; Andrea Hyatt; Kate O'Laughlin; Ann Kennedy; Jamie Prall-Kaliher; Cynthia Jackson; Kris Chambers; Julie Davis; Johnny Johnson, MD; Eric Heitman; Phillip Parrott, Zee Heitman, and Cathy Richard. I cannot extend enough thanks to the many women I have had the privilege of meeting and who have contributed invaluable information and insight. Each of you in your own way wrote this book, and I thank you.

—SB

Thanks are due to Stephanie DeGraff Bender for the opportunity to work on this project; to Barbara Moulton for sage advice and for leading us to Caroline Pincus, our wonderful editor; to Christine Macgenn Rodgerson for astute guidance, deep knowledge of the subject, encouragement, and keen wit; to Ladan Rafii for thoughtful reading and recommendations; to EBHS friends Jan Kaplan Golden and Bette Bayer Schenkel, RPh, for sharing personal stories and professional expertise; to June Casagrande for brilliance and speed in solving many of my writing dilemmas; to Lindsay Berman for insight on style; and to David and Christopher, for appearing regularly in my office while I wrote this book to make sure I didn't forget about really important things, like dinner.

—TC

# MARK YOUR CALENDAR FOR TEN DAYS FROM NOW

Take a look at your calendar and circle the date or put a reminder in your smartphone for ten days from now. Between now and then, you're going to find relief from your perimenopause or menopause symptoms and simply change your life for the better. That's right. Over the next ten days, you will discover how to renew your energy, lift your mood, spend more restful nights, improve your libido, savor foods that make you feel good, sharpen your wits, and brighten up your overall appearance. You'll build stamina with the right mix of exercise, and you'll increase your heart and bone strength.

And if all the noise and confusion about hormone replacement therapy (HRT) has alarmed you, take a deep breath. We've sorted and sifted our way through the medical literature so you don't have to. After all, what busy woman has time for the medical degree she'd need to fully understand the pros and cons of HRT? This should make it a whole lot easier for you to make choices about taking or not taking medication.

*Impossible,* you might think. Do all that in ten days? Possible.

The advice in this guide is simple and straightforward, following the latest science on women's health. We've seen so many women try to navigate this change without a lot of help, and they nearly tear their hair out in the process. That's precisely why we wrote this book.

As women "of a certain age," we are the ultimate multitaskers—organizing and engineering our job and family responsibilities; helping our kids, stepkids, and grandkids along their path; caring for aging relatives; offering community service as volunteers; and negotiating and navigating our marriages, relationships, and friendships. But we shouldn't have to enroll in medical school, leaf through a dozen books, or consult multiple websites to piece together how to handle hot flashes, mood swings, memory lapses, dwindling libido, or other midlife symptoms that are interfering with life.

With each day in this book, you'll find new hints to help you look and feel better. The tenth day caps with an exploration of your spiritual health, so that it, too, flourishes and you can move through your days feeling centered and in control.

For Stephanie, writing this guide feels a bit like coming full circle, which is particularly poignant. Thirty years ago, she founded Full Circle Women's Health, a women's health clinic in Boulder, Colorado, with the philosophy of blending the mental and physical aspects of women's health. At the time, her children were elementary school students ages eight and ten, playing with their beloved action figures and tearing around on their bikes. The term *premenstrual syndrome* (PMS) was only just beginning to be understood. Now her children are grown, with children of their own, and she is a grandmother who has gone through the menopausal transition too. She shares her own experiences here as well as those of the thousands of women she has met through Full Circle Women's Health and in cities all over the United States, where she speaks and gives women's health seminars.

Back in 1982, there was very little information about the ways in which hormones affect women's bodies and psyches, and hormone-related symptoms accompanying the menstrual cycle were dismissed as signs of weakness, self-indulgence, or worse—mental instability. Indeed, we have come a long way since those days. Stephanie has worked with thousands of women who were suffering from PMS, postpartum depression, and later in their lives, symptoms of perimenopause and menopause. On a societal level, there is certainly a greater understanding of women's hormonal health, but she still encounters women on a daily basis who are looking for help and information.

While it's decidedly a good thing that there is a wealth of information on women's hormonal health now, for some women approaching menopause, this information glut has given rise to a new problem—sorting it all out can seem overwhelming. Stephanie's previous books on PMS and perimenopause offered breakthrough information on topics that were rarely acknowledged, let alone discussed. Now Stephanie encounters women who are entering perimenopause or have reached menopause and are experiencing very uncomfortable symptoms, but they're frightened by what they've heard about the harms of HRT. Often, they mistakenly believe that they just have to tough out their symptoms, fearing that HRT is too dangerous and that nothing else works.

We wrote this guide to let women know that their choices are not starkly divided between equally unfavorable options, and to provide manageable, positive steps we can all take to improve this part of our lives. Whether you're in your forties and in perimenopause, meaning that you still have periods although they may be irregular now, or if you're in your forties, fifties, or sixties and have stopped menstruating but still experience menopause symptoms, you'll find help in these pages.

We were recently interested—and amused—to read that anthropologists have discovered that a surprising 25 percent of our Neanderthal sisters lived past the age of forty, contrary to earlier evidence of a far shorter life span. Scientists don't know if these elderly Neanderthal women went through menopause, but reading the article made us speculate about how our experiences compare today, forty thousand years later. Did forty-something Neanderthal women toss off their animal skins in the cave when night sweats came on? Did they feel unexplained sorrow or fatigue without the language to articulate these emotions? We can't know, of course, but we do know today that women experience menopause in distinct ways.

What do you know about your mother's experience of menopause? Perhaps you're reaching menopause at roughly the same age as your mother and with many of the same symptoms. Or your menopausal transition may be completely distinct from hers—with entirely different or more severe symptoms. Maybe you don't know what your mother went through and she isn't here any longer, so you can't ask.

Regardless of which is true for you, this is definitely not your mother's menopause. As a woman reaching menopause today, you have more information about your body, a wider array of choices on what to do, and greater license to be open about your physical, emotional, and spiritual health. Thankfully, we no longer live in a time when women are routinely loaded up with high doses of estrogen to "treat" menopause, a risky practice that has been abandoned. Other women of our mothers' era thought they were toughing it out alone and doing just fine, but many were self-medicating with generous lashings of chardonnay, scotch, or cigarettes. Others resorted to an array of tranquilizers or diet pills that may have kept them thin but jittery or foggy. Some of the symptoms of menopause may be timeless, but your focus on self-care for the next ten days will depart from any dated notions of how women are supposed to think and feel about this time in their lives.

Among sisters, aunts, friends, and cousins who have very similar menopause symptoms, the way they experience them and how much or how little they are bothered by these symptoms can be as varied as their background and appearance. One woman's weight gain may make her feel depressed and out of control, while another woman may accept her more generous waist size and not let it bother her. Night sweats and interrupted sleep can be what sends some women off the rails, while others find that sudden bouts of anxiety, irritability, and/or depression are the menopause symptoms that are hardest to deal with. You may find it useful to inventory your menopause symptoms. What concerns you the most? What do you most want to improve? Write down your thoughts and remember today as the date that you took the first step toward changing the way you look and feel.

There's no right way to go through menopause. But as women, we often get swept up in the millrace of others' needs and neglect our own. Resist that pattern as you pay full attention to your own health and well-being now, and in following this simple, ten-day plan, put yourself first, perhaps for the first time in your life. Tuck this guide into your purse or briefcase, or keep it on your nightstand, and make these health hints your priority for the next week and a half. You've earned this time and consideration.

You can use this guide in one of two ways, but whichever you choose, be sure to follow it for the full ten days. It's easy and effective to follow it chronologically, but if one set of symptoms feels most bothersome to you, feel free to start with the hints for that day. For example, if hot flashes are troubling you more than mood shifts, you may want to begin with the hints for Day 8, "Moisture," and then return to Day 2, "Mood," and then follow the rest of the program in order. Whether you decide to follow the program chronologically for ten days or to create a ten-day sequence that fits your needs, here's what we can tell you for sure: you'll feel better. Check off each tip as you do it, and we guarantee you'll say, "That made me feel good!" every time.

As always, women's stories contribute to our shared knowledge and support. Please post a comment at *www. endyourmenopausemisery.com*, and tell us your story after you finish this ten-day program. We're eager to hear what worked best for you.

# MOOD

The pall that settles without warning. The flash of irritation that turns a routine conversation with a coworker or family member into a heated exchange. Gnawing anxiety that lingers even after a momentary source of stress has been resolved. Bouts of tears that come on unexpectedly. Sound familiar?

Women experience these mood changes during menopause individually. For some, the seesawing nature of their moods—feeling okay one minute and angry, blue, or nervous the next—gives life an unsettled, unpredictable feel that can be unnerving. Other women experience less abrupt shifts in mood but describe an ongoing "flat" feeling or a sense of joylessness where nothing ignites a spark of excitement, enthusiasm, or happiness.

Let's look at how and why these mood changes occur. Estrogen strongly influences the production, transmission, and uptake of key brain chemicals that regulate your mood. As estrogen levels decline steeply during the menopausal years, the complex interplay between this hormone and others like serotonin, dopamine, norepinephrine, and acetylcholine in the brain can alter your mood unpredictably.

As ovaries retire from their job of producing progesterone, the absence of this calming hormone can manifest as increased anxiety or irritability. Women who report feeling especially well during pregnancy are feeling the effects of high progesterone levels that support the growing baby. When ovulation stops, progesterone levels drop nearly to zero.

Hormones don't govern our feelings or behaviors entirely, but they wield considerable clout, especially during menopause. That's important to remember when a shift in mood takes over without any rhyme or reason—you're not suddenly becoming unable to cope.

So don't worry. Even if lately you've felt like you're losing it, there's plenty you can do to prevent these disconcerting mood shifts or minimize their disruptiveness. First, take this short quiz to identify which aspects of your mood changes have been the most bothersome to you in the last three to six months. This will help you clarify the triggers and decide what you'd like to change.

Which statements reflect your feelings?

1. In menopause, I have recaptured my youth. I feel like I am revisiting toddler years, that is, because even a slight irritation can make me feel like I want to fling myself to the floor, drum my heels, and wail.

2. I alternate between wondering, What's wrong with me? and asking myself, What's wrong with all these people who persist in annoying the hell out of me?

3. If anxiety were an Olympic sport, I would go for the gold medal in fretting about past events, worrying about my current circumstances, and getting myself into a tailspin about things that might happen.

4. Menopause has brought about a distinct failure in other people's ability to drive the way I expect them to. While this is intensely irritating, I have built up my arm and jaw muscles by gripping the steering wheel and clenching my teeth.

5. Activities or hobbies that once brought me joy either don't interest me much now or I lack the energy to do them.

6. I swing between feeling deeply justified in roaring at a family member or snapping at a coworker, and later feeling horrified and remorseful about the anger I displayed.

7. I sometimes feel that my best days are behind me.

8. I sometimes feel that my behind's best days are behind me.

9. If outsized tissues for crying jags were available, say somewhere between the size of a hand towel and a bath towel, I would buy several boxes to keep on hand.

10. Things that once lifted my spirits, like wine, sweets, or shopping, either don't work so well anymore or sometimes make me feel worse.

# End Mood Misery

Tongue in cheek aside, if depression, irritability, anxiety, or all three plague you, try giving it a rest, literally. Improving your mood can start with improving your sleep. Erratic or non-refreshing sleep—inability to fall asleep or stay asleep, waking up too early around two or three a.m., or waking up feeling as tired as if you hadn't slept at all—can wreak havoc with anyone's mood. Even the calmest, happiest, and most even-keeled person can't maintain a sense of serenity without sufficient sleep.

Scientists haven't unraveled all the reasons why women have trouble sleeping during menopause. Hot flashes and night sweats are often fingered as the culprit, but they're only one piece of the sleep puzzle. Along with its feel-good role in moods, the brain chemical serotonin also regulates the sleep-wake cycle. An unwelcome tango between insufficient serotonin levels is implicated in menopausal sleep disturbances by night and dim moods by day.

In menopause, more restful sleep may start with changing your perspective and your sleep patterns. If you go to bed anticipating that you'll be wide awake at three a.m., worrying about everything from the world economy to piles of unfinished work on your desk, start telling yourself before you go to bed that you're going to get as much rest as you can.

You've probably read and heard dozens of times that it's important to prepare for sleep, but do you really do it? Today is the day to start your sleep warm-up routine. Begin by making noon your cut-off point for anything with caffeine. Alcohol or exercise right before sleep will only rile you up, so if you have that glass of wine with dinner, finish it at least three hours before you're going to go to bed. A walk after dinner or gentle yoga stretches in the evening can help promote sleep, but it's best to avoid vigorous exercise in the evening. Morning is the best time for that, as you'll read on Day 7.

If it's feasible to rearrange your bedroom and place the bed on the opposite wall for a change, do it. Even a slightly different environment can help to change a disrupted sleep pattern. If your room is noisy, you can reduce sound with a thicker carpet or rug, a soundproof panel on the bottom of your bedroom door, a tapestry hung on the wall to absorb noise, heavier curtains or drapes, and caulking around your windows to limit outside noise. You can also wear earplugs while you sleep, although not everyone likes the idea of not being able to hear while sleeping.

Is the overall ambiance of your room restful? You may want to soften the lighting and choose some new bedding in soothing colors. Silk sheets aren't an indulgence or a luxury—in menopause they may help you sleep better by minimizing dampness from hot flashes or night sweats. Test your mattress and consider whether it's time for a new one. If yours is still in good shape, adding a pillow-top cover can make it even more comfortable.

Think about making your bedroom an electronic-free zone, with no laptop, smartphone, or TV within reach. That helps you avoid scanning that last website or cramming in that last text message before you try to close your eyes. If you read before bed, choose something inspirational or humorous. Keep a selection from your favorite humor writers or inspirational leaders on your nightstand. The latest research shows that sleep not only helps with memory, but that we also continue to learn while we sleep. Make your last "lesson" before bed something that focuses your mind on tranquility or lets you laugh. You'll keep learning how to be calmer or more lighthearted as you sleep.

When insomnia persists, use the time. Awake at three a.m.? Rather than lying in bed worrying about how tired you'll be tomorrow or churning any family or work dilemmas in your mind, get up. Take a blanket or whatever you need to get comfortable into another room. Read, listen to soft music, knit or sew, write or sketch—do anything you enjoy. During daylight, a stolen hour or so to do something like this would be a luxury. Granted, being awake isn't necessarily your first choice, but sometimes it works best not to fight your body when it won't do what you want. When you're feeling sleepy, go back to bed.

Now we come to snoring, which can be a new and troublesome issue in menopause. With less estrogen, the soft muscle tissue in your palate isn't as firm as it once was. In some women, this means more snoring, which can disrupt your sleep (or your partner's).

Sleep apnea occurs more frequently and severely in menopausal women, according to a University of Toronto study that compared sleep patterns in pre- and postmenopausal women. Shifting hormone levels are believed to be behind the increase in this sleep disorder, which produces pauses in breathing or shallow breaths during sleep. These pauses can last from seconds to minutes and may occur from five to thirty times an hour. When breathing starts again, there is often a snorting, choking, or gasping sound. Women with sleep apnea do not get restful sleep, and they wake up feeling tired.

Diagnosing sleep apnea generally involves a sleep study, where you sleep for one night at a sleep laboratory while your breathing, heart rate, and brain waves are monitored. Sleep apnea treatment may include using a continuous positive airway pressure (CPAP) device. A CPAP keeps consistent air gently blowing into your airways to keep them open and to prevent the breathing pauses. Some women find the CPAP mask uncomfortable or the noise from the machine irritating, but there are many good options available now (including much, much quieter machines than previously), and we think you'll be amazed at the double benefit—your own much-improved sleep and your partner's too, if you have one.

Sleeping on your side, rather than on your back, may also help. Some people recommend sewing a tennis ball into your nightgown to prevent you from rolling over on your back, but that seems downright silly. Seriously? Try wedging a pillow up against your back instead—long, narrow body pillows are available for just this purpose. They avoid the problem of how to launder a nightgown with a tennis ball in it.

Alcohol before bed also seems to worsen snoring and sleep apnea, so remember that a nightcap may send you off to sleep briefly only to interrupt your rest during the night. Keeping your weight in a normal range can also help ease snoring. And you may find that elevating your head slightly with an extra pillow or wedge can help you breathe—and sleep—better. If these techniques aren't enough to help with snoring, talk with your dentist. A special mouthpiece is available to guard against snoring, but it must be fitted by a professional.

Changing the way you think about sleep and preparing for sleep just as you would get ready for an important appointment can go a long way toward easing menopausal mood swings during the day and strengthening your ability to manage the emotional changes you may feel.

## Menopause: The Blue Period

If you've found that depression has come along with menopause, you have lots of company. Estimates on the number of women who report feeling depressed in the menopausal years range from 11 to 33 percent, but the numbers may be even higher. Many women may not report their depression or seek help for it but instead try to tough it out. They may feel embarrassed or even ashamed of being depressed, thinking that they have no real serious life issues or crises that merit depression and that they are therefore not entitled to feel the way they do. They may scold or criticize themselves while concealing their vague, general sadness.

Other women may gradually become resigned to feeling flat or indifferent, but you don't have to adapt to a state of tedium.

Hormones strongly influence these feelings during depression. But it can be difficult to sort out how much of the blues is due to estrogen decline and attendant low serotonin levels, and how much results from life changes that tend to come fast and hard during menopause.

There's plenty of nonsense out there suggesting that we poor old menopausal biddies just can't cope with the loss of our youth and fertility or our children leaving home— don't buy into that for a minute. You haven't gotten this far in life without being able to handle whatever life has put in front of you, and that ability doesn't go away during menopause.

Remember that sadness is a normal response to some of what we face in menopause. Our roles as daughters and mothers may shift profoundly. Sometimes women in midlife become the mothers to their mothers, due to frailty, dementia, or loneliness after the death of their fathers. This revised position in the family can contribute to sadness, fatigue, and anxiety. If this phase in your life includes new responsibilities for your mother or other older relatives, the care and support you provide to yourself will greatly increase your ability to help them.

And midlife is the period when many women lose their mothers. Whether the relationship was ideal or fraught with problems, the loss is life changing. If you are coping with menopausal symptoms at the same time that you are adjusting to a world without your mother, your self-care becomes doubly important as you grieve.

Keep fond memories of your mother alive by wearing something of hers, lighting a candle for her, or making one of her favorite recipes. Write down some of your mother's favorite expressions in a notebook, which you can pass along to one of your children or a niece or nephew as part of your family history. Reconcile difficult aspects of your relationship with your mother by writing her a letter or listing three or four things you learned from her, even if they are examples of how not to behave.

Telling stories about our mothers can be healing, too, regardless of the relationship. One woman told of going to a silver-polishing party with a group of women around Mother's Day. Each woman was asked to bring a piece of silver or any special object that had belonged to her mother. At the gathering, they polished the objects and told a story about their mothers. Some of the women's mothers were still alive and vigorous, others were in failing health, some had passed on fairly recently, and others long ago. There was a mix of laughter and tears, and the women came away understanding more about themselves, their mothers, and each other.

If you are a mother, the changes that come with menopause frequently coincide—and in some cases clash with—a transformation in the relationship with your children. Perhaps your children are teenagers, so there are days when menopausal irritability and teen sullenness form a particularly combustible mix in the household. If your children are older, you may have a mix of wistfulness and delight as you watch them go out on their own into the world. Or you may find yourself feeling burdened by children who are a bit slower than you would like in leaving the nest, or who continue to rely on you financially when you wish they were paying their own way now.

Remind yourself that you still have the capacity to adjust to life's changes, just as you have in the past. You've done it before, and you can do it again. Being sad doesn't mean you are not being brave or that you can't handle life—you can. Give some careful thought to the degree to which sadness or depression is interfering with your life, and then try these strategies for dealing with it.

## Don't Be Sad Alone

This piece of advice means different things to different women, depending on their personality. Women who take comfort in prayer or another spiritual practice often find solace in asking for their God's presence in their struggle, with a prayer that can be as simple as "God, please be with me in my sadness, worry, fear, or anger." Other women benefit from resolving to pick up the phone when depression threatens to get the best of them. Call someone you miss, whom you haven't talked with in a while, and catch up. Get in touch with a friend whose company you enjoy. Make a plan to do something that makes it impossible to feel sad while you're doing it and that gives you something fun to anticipate—see a funny movie or play, take in an evening of stand-up comedy, attend a concert together, or pick a beautiful place to meet for a walk.

## Decide What to Let Go Of

It's very powerful to decide to limit our suffering about the things we can't change. What are those things in your life? Write them down. Look over the list, and tear it to bits if you like. Then choose whatever ritual you prefer to symbolize letting go of these sources of sadness or stress. Bury the paper pieces in a flowerpot or in your garden. Watch them go up in smoke in your barbecue or fireplace, or stand by while they swirl down the toilet (make sure you've torn the list into tiny enough pieces, so a plumber's bill isn't an additional stress). You might even write your list of things you want to release on a wall, and then paint over it. Or do as one woman did and put them in your deep freeze where they can't live. The unburdening is symbolic but powerful. Anytime you find your mind returning to these causes of stress or sorrow, remind yourself by saying out loud, "I burned that," or "I buried that." Visualize it as gone, over, done, with no more power over your life. You're in charge.

## Get a Move On

Menopause was once discreetly referred to as "the change of life," usually in a lowered tone and generally not in mixed company. Remember that "going through the change" doesn't necessarily have to be all about hot flashes or feeling wistful for times gone by. Take stock of your personal and professional relationships. Which support your happiness and which impede it? Deciding to move on or limit your interaction with people who don't bring anything positive to your life doesn't have to involve confrontation or acrimony—it means you make the choice to emphasize the people and things that boost your spirits and make you feel good. Write down the names of people who are welcome in your life.

## Work It Out

Reflect on your work and its role in your satisfaction or, conversely, in your stress or depression. In rocky economic times, there's a not-so-subtle undercurrent in many work settings that we place our foreheads in the dust to express gratitude that we have a job at all. Yes, many of us may not have the option of leaving a job now, but we can refashion the work we're doing. Take a class to boost your knowledge and talk with your supervisor about adjusting your role. If you're currently facing the stress of seeking work, look into volunteering for an organization that can benefit from your professional skills. Organizations that serve children, seniors, and veterans are always looking for help. Or if you have a friend who owns a business, see if you can help out as a temp or a volunteer.

## Face Sadness and Fear

We can spend valuable time and energy fighting what we're feeling or trying to run from sadness, regret, or anxiety. Accepting a feeling doesn't mean you're stuck with it. But there may be times when the antidote to stress or despondency is telling yourself that you're going to live with it for a specific amount of time. You decide how long that will be—the next hour, afternoon, or day—and then you're going to either set it aside as something that can't be fixed or as something you'll face again when you're ready.

## Count Your Blessings, Set Down Your Burdens

Many women find it affirming to make a daily note of three things they are grateful for that day. Keep a notebook by your bed just for this purpose. Take your pick from the large and small things that grace your life—a colleague who gave you a hand today, a grandchild's gummy grin, your health, the wisecracking friend who never fails to make you laugh—the people and things you would dearly miss if they were not present in your life but that were there today. Doing this each evening and leafing through this notebook at times when life seems dreary can increase your optimism, which positively impacts your health. Research shows that taking the time to place yourself in a state of gratitude lowers stress levels and may heighten immune function. What are three things you are grateful for right now? Occasionally, take the daily notebook one step further and send someone you've named on your gratitude list a card, note, or email to say, "Thank you!"

## Reach Out to Help Someone, and Help Yourself

Sometimes the best way to shake a persistent cloud of unhappiness is to give someone else a hand. In your neighborhood, among your colleagues, or in your circle of friends, there's always any number of people whose day you can brighten immeasurably, whether it's a single parent struggling to do it all, someone who simply needs a friend, a neighbor going through cancer treatment, or a friend who recently lost a family member. Your gift to that person or family can be a phone call to let them know you're thinking of them, offering to give them a ride or to pick up groceries, walking their dog, or dropping off an evening meal. They will be touched by your empathy and thoughtfulness, and you'll find that turning your focus to someone who needs help will exchange your feelings of sadness or anxiety for a sense of satisfaction at having made a difference.

## Breathe

Many menopausal women describe an unsettling shift of mood that seems to come on without warning, in the car, at the desk, or lying awake at night—a sudden surge of anxiety or despair often accompanied by a sprinting heart rate or sweaty, light-headed sensation. That's a great time to do a breathing exercise.

You can do this simple breathing exercise anytime, anywhere to slow down your heart rate and deepen your breathing until the uncomfortable feeling lifts. Take a deep breath in and, as you do so, say or think, "Breathe in peace,"

"Breathe in relaxation," or "Breathe in serenity." Breathe in slowly through your nostrils for a count of four, and then slowly breathe out for a count of four. As you breathe out, say or think, "Breathe out the nervousness," or "Breathe out the gloom," or "Breathe out the worry." Picture the anxiety or discontent leaving your body with each long, slow exhale, replaced by peace and calm with each inhale.

There's a certain irony in the fact that the National Center for Telehealth & Technology, a division of the US Department of Defense, has a smartphone app to guide you through relaxation breathing. You can find it at *www. t2health.org/apps/breathe2relax*. It's effective, and you can customize it to suit your pace. But is being tethered to smartphones and computers to the point where we're relying on them to teach us how to relax necessarily a great thing? What do you think? Please leave your comments at *www.endyourmenopausemisery.com*.

## Ask for Help

When family or work responsibilities threaten to overwhelm you, send up a flare. For some women, this means having to relinquish a former notion of themselves as entirely self-sufficient, or as the one everyone else comes to for help, not the one asking for assistance. Handing off some of your duties can make the difference between feeling frazzled and stressed, and having a moment to yourself. Decide what you need and make your requests direct and specific. No vague, "I don't know what to have for dinner,"

"The house is a mess," "I have so many invoices to do," or "I need to go check on Mom." It's way too easy for family, friends, siblings, or colleagues to ignore hazy statements like these. Swap them for clear requests for help: "Will you please bring home takeout or stop by the market for milk?" "Will you please (fill in what you need here—vacuum, fold the laundry, change the sheets, pick up the living room, do half this pile of invoices)?" "Could you please drive over to Mom's and see that she's okay and ask if she needs anything?" You'll find that asking for help isn't so hard after you've done it a few times, and when you let your family, friends, or colleagues know how much you appreciate their help, you give them a gift too.

## Change the Venue, and Make the Change of Pace a Literal One

Get outside to lift your spirits. Instead of a coffee or lunch date, make a walk date and pick a new venue, a different park, lake, beach, or trail where you can walk and talk. Try the opposite of a power walk occasionally—change the pace and move more deliberately so you can listen, smell, touch, and observe what's around you. Maya Angelou said, "A bird doesn't sing because it has an answer, it sings because it has a song." Go outside and replenish your well as you listen to birdsong, feel the sun pour in, hear the wind rustle or the rain fall if you like it, and breathe in the scent of the water or flowers. You'll feel as the great naturalist John Muir did when he said, "The sun-love made me strong."

But not all mood changes in midlife need to disquiet us. We can also feel grateful that the uncertainty and insecurity we may have felt as younger women now gives way to a more reflective and discerning way of regarding the world, and a certain sageness in viewing ourselves. Our wisdom—some hard earned, some gently and slowly acquired over time—can be trusted to serve us well as we experience menopause.

# MEMORY

Former poet laureate Billy Collins gives a delightful view of memory loss in his poem "Forgetfulness."

> *The name of the author is the first to go*
> *followed obediently by the title, the plot,*
> *the heartbreaking conclusion, the entire novel*
> *which suddenly becomes one you have never read, never*
> *even heard of,*
>
> *as if, one by one, the memories you used to harbor*
> *decided to retire to the southern hemisphere of the*
> *brain,*
> *to a little fishing village where there are no phones.*
>
> *Long ago you kissed the names of the nine Muses good-*
> *bye*
> *and watched the quadratic equation pack its bag,*
> *and even now as you memorize the order of the planets,*

*something else is slipping away, a state flower perhaps,*

*the address of an uncle, the capital of Paraguay.*

*Whatever it is you are struggling to remember*

*it is not poised on the tip of your tongue,*

*not even lurking in some obscure corner of your spleen.*

*It has floated away down a dark mythological river*

*whose name begins with an L as far as you can recall,*

*well on your own way to oblivion where you will join those*

*who have even forgotten how to swim and how to ride a bicycle.*

*No wonder you rise in the middle of the night*

*to look up the date of a famous battle in a book on war.*

*No wonder the moon in the window seems to have drifted*

*out of a love poem that you used to know by heart.*

*"Forgetfulness" from* Questions About Angels,
*by Billy Collins, © 1991. Reprinted by
permission of the University of Pittsburgh Press.*

Today is the day you can ease your alarm about sudden memory gaps and quiet your fear that you're on the cusp of dementia. Changes in memory and concentration at midlife are very common, but you don't have to live with them. You can improve your memory and mental sharpness with simple activities and routines you'll enjoy. And on Day 6, you'll also learn about choosing foods to support your memory.

As in mood, the twin problems of declining estrogen and lack of sleep conspire to produce the troubling "foggy" state so many women describe during menopause. Your brain—that three-pound powerhouse that controls everything you think and do—has estrogen receptors in many of its structures, notably the hippocampus. Central to memory and learning, the hippocampus has equal parts on the right and left sides of the brain. Estrogen also affects the circuitry in the prefrontal cortex, which interacts with the medial temporal lobe where the hippocampus is located. With less estrogen to promote the release of acetylcholine and other brain chemicals, the process of transmitting information between nerve cells on both sides of the brain can suffer. The interruption in these nerve pathways can make you feel like your brain is sputtering when you're trying to concentrate or remember something.

Remember that certain age-related memory changes are normal. If you can't find your keys or glasses, you draw a complete blank on someone's name, or you wander into a room and then have no idea why you went there or what you were looking for, you don't need to fret. These memory changes can be irritating, but they don't signal the onset of progressive, worsening memory loss. If lapses in memory or cognition begin to interfere with your ability to function, it's time to see your doctor. Examples of these would include being unable to follow a recipe or balance a checkbook; feeling disoriented about the date, time, or season; or showing impaired judgment by giving money away to someone you don't know or by appearing in public in your pajamas.

Here are some straightforward tips you can use to help bring your memory out of retirement from that little fishing village.

### Rest Your Brain

Review what you learned on Day 2 about improving your sleep and make sure you're allocating enough time for rest. If you're trying to do every last thing you can in the evening, that accomplishment may actually shortchange you the next day. When you're sleeping, you're not merely resting your muscles and bones—your brain keeps sorting and storing information. Inadequate sleep makes it more difficult for you to perform memory-related tasks: everything from recalling words or names to being on top of what goes in that quarterly report you've prepared dozens of times before.

### Plan to Review Your Medications at Your Next Doctor Visit

Your prescription or over-the-counter medication may play a role in blurring the edges of your memory. If you regularly take an antihistamine to control allergy-related sniffles or an antacid to calm your stomach, be aware that some of these medications interfere with the activity of acetylcholine in your brain. Certain antidepressants and antispasmodic drugs may also disrupt cognitive function. If you're among the approximately 20 million Americans who take a cholesterol-lowering statin drug, changes in your memory could be linked to the medication, according to anecdotal evidence. Medication-related changes in memory or cognition are often mild enough that it may not have occurred to you to associate a fuzzy memory with any medication you're taking. That's why it's a good idea to check in with your doctor to review your medications. You can discuss whether it's possible to discontinue taking any of your medications or if a change to another medication or dosage will lessen memory-related side effects.

## Savor a Bit of Dark Chocolate Every Day

A study published in *Physiology and Behavior* shows that the flavanols in dark chocolate boost blood flow to the brain, improving recall and visual performance. Have your dose of chocolate memory medicine any way you like it—make cocoa or chocolate milk with dark chocolate, enjoy a scoop of chocolate ice cream, or let a morsel of dark chocolate melt on your tongue. If you prefer savory to sweet, make or buy mole sauce made with dark chocolate and put it on chicken, rice, or vegetables. If you enjoy about an ounce of dark chocolate daily, you'll reap the benefits without piling on excess sugar, calories, or fat. If you prefer to stay away from chocolate, cocoa supplements offer the flavanols without the fat or sugar, too, but also without the fun.

## Hike to Bolster the Hippocampus

New research shows that the hippocampus portion of the brain, the memory storehouse, increases in size with regular aerobic exercise, even among people who had been previously sedentary. MRI brain images of study participants showed increased volume in the hippocampus among the aerobic exercise group. You can meet the twin goals of boosting memory and keeping fit in menopause with thirty minutes of daily walking. Even women who insist they don't have time to walk can find three ten-minute blocks of time to walk. You can also make your walk a moving meditation by deciding that you'll keep a deliberate pace and use the time to think about a simple affirmation or prayer, such as "I feel really good today," or "Thank you for my health," or "Everything is getting better." Tell yourself, "I'm not going to think about anything negative while I'm walking," and resist the urge to ruminate about work, family, or finances as you walk. All those things will wait while you spend a few minutes building up your hippocampus, strengthening your bones, and evening out your mood. On Day 7, you'll learn more about the overall benefits of exercise in menopause.

## Harness Memory Power Using All Five Senses

You can boost the effectiveness of your to-do lists and smartphone reminders by using the full power of all five senses. If you find that you're lying in bed night after night thinking, *I forgot to call so and so,* concentrate for a moment on the sound of that person's voice. That extra sensory detail can keep you from letting that call slip your mind again. When you need to pick something up from the store—your dark chocolate, perhaps—imagine the taste or smell of whatever it is you need to buy. You can use a visual image of color to help jog your memory, such as envisioning the color of your bank logo to remind you to go online and pay your credit card bill or to mail the check for your godchild's birthday gift. If you find you're losing time and stressing yourself by looking for files, papers, or other objects over and over, engage your sense of touch to help you remember where things are. Along with saying to yourself, "I'm putting this form in the medical insurance file," or "I'm stashing the scissors in the tool drawer," take an extra second to run your hand along the file folder or drawer surface, giving your mind an extra imprint of where you are placing the object. This additional sensory experience will help you recall later when you need to find that paper, gadget, pair of glasses, set of keys, jacket, or purse.

## *Keep Stress in Check to Increase Memory and Concentration*

We all know the feeling of being so rattled that we can scarcely recollect our own name, let alone important details we need to be present at work or at home. Stress is a major offender in memory problems. Don't let rising panic or frustration take over when you can't remember something. Step back, step outside if you can, and practice your breathing exercises. Tell yourself, "It will come to me in a minute." Picture yourself clearing out your mind, emptying it of the things you don't need to think about, and making room for what you want to recall. Your ability to relax lets you enjoy a steady and calm mood, and it also sharpens your ability to recollect.

## Lessen Overload to Help Your Memory

Some research suggests that the foggy feeling many women experience in menopause isn't a matter of being unable to remember but instead reflects difficulty learning new information, or encoding it in your brain. Women who lament feeling less sharp or alert when they reach menopause haven't become less intelligent or less able to learn, but assimilating new information may take a bit longer because it's simply become harder to keep track of everything. The glut of memories you have stored begin to interfere with each other. Are you the repository for information about everyone's deadlines, appointments, health care, meal schedules, transportation, babysitting, clothing, whereabouts, birthdays, anniversaries, and more? Are you juggling the needs of parents, partner, pets, kids, boss, colleagues, and neighbors? Think about what you can set aside and decide what you no longer need to keep track of at work and at home. Do you call family members to remind them to call other family members on their birthday? You don't need to take on responsibility for everyone else's memory bank.

Following these hints will help you recall what's important and will ease your anxiety about those momentary wobbles in your memory. Trust that you'll recall what you need to remember, even if it takes a few extra seconds. And be aware that when something slips your mind, it might be nature's gentle hint that you don't need to be in charge of every detail.

# MIRROR

Sometimes it's the mirror that delivers the shock; sometimes it's a photo. Changes in skin, hair, and muscle tone show up during the menopausal transition and can bring an unwelcome sense that our attractive years are over. This isn't true. Today you will get going on a series of tips and tricks to look your best while you continue with what you learned about feeling your best on Days 1, 2, and 3.

Comedian Lily Tomlin jokes that she needs a "wattlectomy" to correct the midlife folds in her neck. In an episode of *The Golden Girls*, Dorothy laments new and unwanted facial hair, plaintively telling Blanche and Rose, "One day I woke up, and I had a little beard." These quips make us laugh and cringe at the same time, but we don't have to surrender to having our looks being the butt of jokes. Even with more lines on your face or more gray threading through your hair, you can thrive and shine as you go through menopause; it just takes a little effort and some different techniques. Read on for advice on creating a makeover.

# Invest in Your Looks, and Believe You're Worth It

A new phase in life and changing body contours mean your look and style may need to take a different shape during menopause. Even if you've favored a consistent style of clothing, a usual haircut, the same cosmetics, or standard jewelry because they have worked for years, they may not be the right choices for you now. In fact, this consistency can contribute to a feeling of boredom and drabness. Today you are going to assess what you have in your closet, jewelry box, and makeup bag, and make some decisions about what stays and what goes. At the same time, make the commitment right now to swap out the old for some new. You'll breathe new life into your image in the mirror.

## Clear Your Closet—It's Cathartic

Whether your closet is a riot of clothes and shoes; a neatly organized, color-coordinated system; or somewhere in the middle, start at one end and go through each item of clothing.

Make three piles:

1. Keep

2. Rehabilitate

3. Donate

"It was expensive," "I've had it a long time," and "I wear it a lot" are not automatic criteria for designating something for the Keep pile. Decide to keep only those clothes that you feel good wearing and that can be paired with lots of other clothes for variety. Your Rehabilitate pile may include pieces that can be tailored or trimmed anew. Can a shirt, jacket, or pants be lengthened, shortened, taken in, or let out? If you're on a budget, alterations are frequently less expensive than buying something new.

Make a trip to the antique store for vintage buttons to enliven a jacket, or to the fabric store for lace or colorful textile borders to bedeck the hem of a skirt or pants. And if crafts or sewing aren't your thing, or if you're not inclined to have a tailor refurbish any of your clothes, don't feel guilty. Put the clothes you aren't going to wear into the Donate pile. Choose a women's shelter, hospital thrift store, or other charity in your community that either sells clothing to raise funds or provides clothing to people in need.

## Jettison the Old Jewelry

Have a jar of jewelry cleaning solution at the ready and sort through your baubles. Sometimes a dip in the jewelry cleaner is enough to give a ring, earrings, or pin the sparkle and shine of something new. If you've been holding on to pieces that were your mother's, aunt's, or grandmother's, but you never wear them, now may be the time to pass them on to a daughter or niece. Write down a brief story about the piece—"Uncle Jack brought this locket from Paris," "Mom always wore this pin at Christmastime," or "These earrings came from the department store downtown

that is long gone, where Nana used to take me for tea"—
and put it in the box or bag with the jewelry you give away.
This way you pass along a memory too. It's great to donate
costume jewelry. If you have girls younger than ten in your
neighborhood, they might be ecstatic to have your beads
and bangles for dress-up. If you'd rather not give jewelry
away, think about selling whatever you no longer wear to a
reputable antique store or jeweler.

## Sift Through Your Shoes

One woman joked that she sorted her shoes into Keep
and What Was I Thinking? piles. Take a look at your shoe
stock. If you have multiple pairs with only a slight variation
on the same theme, keep only the most comfortable pairs
and those in the best shape. Anything you haven't worn in
a year, let go. The same applies to any shoes that induce
wincing when you walk. Simplifying your closet is part of
simplifying your life, and you'll make room for new things.

## Going for Something New

Now it's time for the fun part, which is choosing new
clothes, shoes, and accessories to replace some of the pieces
you donated. The first rule of fashion for mature women is:
there are no rules. Well, maybe one, and that is: wear what's
comfortable, looks stylish, and makes you feel great. If
you've chosen the same styles over the years, consider asking
a personal shopper at a department store or a salesperson

at a boutique for help in selecting some different textures, designs, and colors. Check in your community for consignment or thrift shops, too, where you can often find good quality, scarcely worn clothing for very reasonable prices.

Go with a sister or trusted friend for some feedback and perspective, and let the salesperson know that you're interested in supplementing the essentials of a mix-and-match wardrobe that can work for more than one season. Think about smoothing out the edges—keep warm with soft sweaters rather than boxy jackets, for example. Dressing in layers makes it easy for you to peel off a cardigan when a hot flash hits. Select pants, a skirt, or a dress you can wear often and pair with multiple tops or jackets, and think beyond black as a basic color. Emphasize quality rather than quantity, especially when you're choosing some new shoes or a new bag. Really good shoes and bags will last for years.

If you're thinking there's no room in the budget for a wardrobe makeover, take a good look at every line item to see what you can shift or reallocate. If there's a bill or service you can get rid of or pare down so that you can buy some new frocks, go ahead and make that fiscal decision. You deserve to look good and feel well, and you're worth the money.

## Every Day Is a Good Hair Day

It's true that menopause may bring more than the usual share of bad hair days, as the dip in hormone levels can cause hair to become thinner or to lose luster. But you can eat to help restore bounce and shine to your hair—we'll learn about those foods tomorrow, and today we'll focus on minimum hair maintenance for maximum style and ease.

Less may be more when it comes to coloring, styling, and shampooing your hair at this stage of life. Your hair is producing less oil now and may not need to be washed more than twice a week. If it seems hard to break a lifelong habit of more frequent shampooing, try it for a couple of weeks and see how you like it. Your hair may actually be less flyaway if it is washed less often, and you certainly will save time and hair product costs. Try a volumizing shampoo if your hair has become thinner, and add a bit of gel for more body.

Take time to condition your hair at least once a week. If you generally shampoo, condition, and rinse in rapid succession so that you can scramble out of the shower and get on to the next thing, try slowing down. Put the conditioner in your hair, get out of the shower, and wrap your hair in a warm towel. Leave the conditioner in for ten or fifteen minutes, and while you're waiting for it to moisturize and smooth your hair, do something relaxing—sit by a sunny window, read a magazine, have a cup of tea, or just sink into a comfortable chair with your feet up and your eyes closed. This mini-break helps your hair and your psyche.

# The Gray Area

If you've already been coloring your hair for years or have recently reached the stage where there is more gray threading your hair than ever before, today is the day to stop and assess. Do you want or need to cover the silver? Salt and pepper can be gorgeous just as it is, or a few highlights can bring out some blonde while lowlights can freshen up darker hair. Camouflage isn't obligatory as we get older and, in some cases, hair color achieves the opposite effect, giving a harsher, more severe look when natural silver or gray may be softer and more flattering.

And if silver isn't for you, that's fine too. Whether you color your hair at home or have it done at a salon, select a color that blends well with your natural look, neither too brassy nor too dark. That saves you the time, effort, and money required to keep up with growing-in roots that show a lot of contrast.

## Cut and Dried

A new hairstyle can lift your spirits and help counter the effects of thinning or lackluster hair. If you've favored the same hairstyle for years, by all means, keep it if you're happy with the way it looks and feels and with the amount of time you need to spend to keep it looking the way you want it. But if you're up for a change, talk with your stylist about a different way to cut and shape your hair so it's comfortable and easy to take care of. If your hair has been short or long consistently, think about going in the opposite direction with a little more or a little less length for a change. Beauty experts agree that there's no relationship between hair length and age—if you're tired of a short and sensible bob and want to grow it out for a change, do it! You can always change it again if it turns out not to be to your liking.

## Hair You'd Rather Not Have

Then there is the matter of other hair during menopause, when seesawing estrogen and testosterone levels can coarsen and thicken facial hair. As estrogen diminishes, the influence of the small amount of testosterone that we continue to produce becomes more prominent. If you notice that hair on your chin, upper lip, and eyebrows has become wirier and seems to sprout with maddening regularity, that's why. Managing bothersome facial hair at home requires a bit of time and a few tools: a precise pair of tweezers with a very good grip to pluck the peskiest hairs; small, very sharp scissors to trim hair closely to the skin on the upper lip or chin areas; and a lighted, magnifying mirror mounted on the bathroom wall.

Cream bleach specifically for facial hair can help lighten and conceal hair, and bleaching doesn't need to be done as frequently as plucking or using depilatory creams for hair removal. If you don't already do it, treat yourself occasionally to having your eyebrows professionally shaped—it gives a smooth, polished look to your face and accentuates your eyes. It also makes it easier for you to keep your brows neat because you have a pattern to follow.

Threading, electrolysis, or waxing can also be used to remove facial hair. At-home waxing kits save money but not necessarily time unless you're skilled at the technique.

Rashes, redness, and breakouts sometimes follow waxing to remove facial hair, so you may want to have a professional do this to minimize the side effects. Some women prefer threading, the centuries-old technique of using cotton thread to lift out hair. Threading requires no chemicals, and some women find it less painful and less expensive than other methods.

Some women are plagued by severe facial hair that requires a prescription medication to control. These medications aren't recommended for routine hair removal, however.

# Skin in the Menopausal Game

The not-so-good news: menopausal hormone changes also contribute to dry, itchy, and thinner-looking skin in many women. Your body takes longer to regenerate new cells, so that healthy glow you once had may seem to have vanished. Less collagen and elastin, which makes your skin pliant, can mean more wrinkles, lines, and sags, and your skin may appear rougher. Sometimes fluctuating hormone levels can trigger breakouts too.

But there's lots of good news: you're going to start taking better care of your skin today, and here is why. Did you know that your skin is your largest organ, and that it is part of your immune system? Taking good care of your skin isn't an indulgence or a vanity—it's a very important part of taking care of your overall health. You can nourish your skin by eating delicious, colorful foods and drinking plenty of water. You'll learn more on Day 7 about how good-looking food on your plate helps create lovely skin. Today, you can rejuvenate your skin with some simple changes in your cleansing and makeup techniques.

Wash your face with a good, moisturizing cleanser and apply a moisturizer with at least SPF 15 to protect your skin from the sun. Skin products with alpha-lipoic acid or retinol can help brighten dull-looking skin, but use products containing alpha hydroxy acids sparingly, as these can be very drying. A moisturizer with a slight tint that matches your skin tone may be all you need to smooth out fine lines. Apply the moisturizer when you first get out of the shower.

Some women apply a makeup primer first (or spackle, as one woman wickedly called it) and allow it to dry before putting on a bit of foundation or tinted moisturizer. The primer can help fill in lines and create a smoother finish. Liquids give a softer look, so it's best to stay away from anything powdery, as powder particles can settle into lines on your face and draw attention to them rather than away from them.

Thinner skin means thinner lips, too, unfortunately, but this is easily fixed by subtly outlining your lips with a soft-colored lip pencil, avoiding dark lipstick, which can make lips look thinner and flatter, and adding a touch of clear or lightly tinted gloss either alone or on top of your lipstick. You can use lip plumpers to puff up your lips, but the ingredients in these products work by irritating the skin on your lips so that they swell slightly in response. Most women in menopause don't need to subscribe to the philosophy that one must suffer to be beautiful, so you can skip anything that makes you feel like you've been stung by a wasp.

Brighten and wake up your eyes with a bit of matte shadow in a neutral color, such as cream or cocoa, that matches your skin tone. Avoid anything shimmery around your eyes because the sparkle can accentuate wrinkles and lines. If you have a very steady hand and can apply a thin stroke of eyeliner just at your lash line before you brush on some soft shadow, this helps to show off the contour of your eye and takes attention away from skin around the eyes that may be sagging. You can also draw attention to your brows with just a hint of color that you apply with a brush or soft pencil. This is a quick, easy eye makeup routine that shows off the natural gleam in your eye while softening the effects of time.

## Create Your Own Spa

Tend to the rest of your skin, too, by massaging your hands and feet with moisturizer regularly—you increase your circulation and give yourself a few extra moments to unwind. Light a candle with a delicious fragrance to set a mood of relaxation. Choose a gentle scrub with a scent that soothes you and apply it all over your body with a soft mitt or loofah. Pay attention to rough areas around your knees, heels, and elbows. You'll glow on the outside from the scrub's refreshing effects, and taking this time for yourself can also help still the chatter in your mind and recharge your energy. This home spa treatment is simple and inexpensive but has valuable benefits.

Treat yourself to the occasional facial, massage, or spa scrub by a professional too. All you need to do is show up. Yes, spa treatments can be pricey, but watch for local discounts and enjoy this pampering without guilt—you're worth it. If you live near a school of massage therapy, you can take advantage of inexpensive massages by students who are completing their training.

## She Has a Beautiful Smile

If your teeth could stand to be a bit brighter, ask your dentist to recommend whitening strips that you can use at home. Go for just enough whiteness to lift the darkening effects of coffee, tea, or wine. Avoid the porcelain look, which can appear artificial and startling.

Choose the skin care and makeup products that match your budget. Remember that reasonably priced products are available, and don't forget to check your kitchen cupboard for natural beauty enhancers. Rinse teabags in warm water and place them on your eyes to reduce puffiness, make your own facial mask with cooked oatmeal mixed with egg white and a bit of honey, use plain old white sugar for a gentle facial scrub, and rub olive oil onto rough or dry spots on your skin. A spray bottle of olive oil makes a very convenient and economical moisturizer. A steep price, celebrity endorsement, or supposedly secret or magical ingredient in any serum or elixir does not necessarily mean a better look for you.

Whether you favor home remedies, minerals, botanicals, or other makeup formulas, your most important cosmetic, the one you absolutely can't do without, is your smile. More than anything you can put on your face, your smile shows the world that you are relaxed, confident, and happy with the way you look.

Consider the words of Bonnie Prudden, the amazing rock climber and fitness expert who lived a vigorous and exciting life until she died at age ninety-seven. She said, "You can't turn back the clock, but you can wind it up again." Looking and feeling marvelous in menopause doesn't mean trying to recapture the way we looked in another decade. It does mean winding up the clock again and going forward with radiance and joy, content with who we are.

# MOJO

Ladies, let's have a show of hands. Given the choice between making love and rolling over to go to sleep, how many of you would prefer shut-eye to sex these days? If you came down on the sleep side of this menopausal straw poll, you're not alone. According to the Sexuality Information and Education Council of the United States (SIECUS), 45 percent of women surveyed said their desire for sex dipped after menopause. Slightly more than one-third said they experienced no change in desire, and 10 percent said their desire had increased. (If we knew what those women were eating or drinking, we'd offer it by the caseload, but we don't, so read on for tips you can use.)

Some women experience a gradual waning of sexual desire over a period of years. Others report a sharp plummet in their need for and enjoyment of sex when they enter menopause or have a hysterectomy. In either instance, this drop in desire prompts mixed emotions in perimenopausal and menopausal women. Feelings you may recognize include:

- **Embarrassment.** Some women say they feel as if they have lost some essential part of themselves when they no longer desire or enjoy sex. They often hesitate to speak up about this change, not breathing a word to their spouse or partner and not mentioning it to their doctor.

- **Wistfulness.** When sleep begins to seem more appealing than a steamy night spent making love, women often say they miss the days of sexual urgency when they couldn't get enough of their husbands and the reverse. They don't know how to rekindle that flame, worry that it's gone forever, and lament that the exciting, sexy time of their life may be behind them.

- **Depression.** Some women equate a drop in sexual desire with a diminishment in their own desirability or attractiveness, and they find this leaves them feeling lost, useless, and depressed. This change often coincides with a profound shift in various roles—as mothers if children are leaving the nest; as daughters if elderly or ill parents require more care or have passed away; and as spouses as years together can give way to boredom, irritation, or both.

These life adjustments, paired with a sense that sex isn't that interesting or pleasurable, can leave women feeling unsexy, blue, and asking themselves, "Who am I now? What is my purpose?"

# Sounds Familiar

Which of these best describes your experience?

I have the urge to have sex:

- ❑ Regularly
- ❑ Less often than I used to
- ❑ Rarely

I notice the following changes in my vaginal tissue that make intercourse uncomfortable or even painful:

- ❑ Dryness
- ❑ Burning
- ❑ Itching
- ❑ Narrowing
- ❑ All of the above

These parts of my body are now less sensitive to erotic touch:

- ❑ Breasts
- ❑ Vagina
- ❑ Clitoris
- ❑ Other

It takes longer for me to become sexually aroused now.

- ❑ Yes
- ❑ No

My experience of orgasm has changed, and now:

- ❏ It takes longer to achieve orgasm.
- ❏ Orgasm is less intense.
- ❏ Painful uterine cramps follow orgasm.
- ❏ Other: _____

Let's take a look at why these changes in sexual desire and response can occur in midlife and, more important, the solutions for recapturing your pleasure.

Vaginal tissue thins and dries out as estrogen levels decline in menopause. In fact, the vagina changes from forty layers of skin to four. This thin, drier tissue is less sensitive and often doesn't lubricate, which can make intercourse feel more like sanding than something sensuous. Hormone shifts may also be responsible for decreased blood flow to the genitals, resulting in slower arousal and decreased sensitivity to touch.

The drop in testosterone is believed to be the culprit in extinguishing the sexual spark that many women report during the menopausal years, although studies don't bear this out. Produced by the adrenal glands and ovaries, testosterone in women falls by as much as 50 percent by the time a woman reaches age forty-five. Interestingly, while some research shows that low testosterone levels in women are not always matched with low libido, women who take testosterone do seem to experience increased sexual desire.

Testosterone is sometimes prescribed off label for low libido, meaning the FDA has not approved its use for this purpose. Low-dose, short-term use may be appropriate for some women, but the type of testosterone and the dosage are very important in order to avoid unwelcome side effects like acne and facial hair. We'll review this option in more depth on Day 9, when we talk about the role of medication in menopause.

## The Good News

Don't believe for a minute that a vibrant and satisfying sex life is elusive once you reach a certain age. Here's how to reclaim the passion you once enjoyed and infuse your intimate life with new ardor.

## Use Your Most Important Sex Organ, Your Mouth

Yes, use your mouth to kiss, lick, nibble, and so on, of course, but more important, use it to talk with your husband or partner about the changes you are experiencing and how you feel. If you've felt hesitant about this, start with simple, short, clear messages: "I'm having hormonal changes." You may want to reassure your spouse that those changes don't affect how you feel about him. Be clear about what you need: "It takes me longer to become aroused now." "I feel good when you (go more slowly, more quickly, touch me here)." Some women find that once erogenous zones, like their breasts, are now not only less sensitive to erotic touch but also that the sensation of touch can be downright irritating. Let your partner know where you like to be touched now—whatever works for you. And when you don't feel like having sex, communicate honestly about that, too, rather than avoiding the issue. It's okay to say, "I'm not feeling like making love right now." Remember that men may experience a lessening sex drive in midlife too.

Here is a communication activity to do together with your partner. It will not only help you think through how you're feeling, but it's also a way of letting your partner know that you're actively seeking to increase your sexual enjoyment. Choose a place where you're relaxed and comfortable, and add any amenities you like: a fire in the fireplace, a shared glass of wine, some candlelight. Take turns reading each question aloud and responding. Be clear with your partner that this is a fun, sexy activity with no right or wrong answers. See what happens!

I prefer making love:

- ❏ In the dark
- ❏ With the lights on
- ❏ By candlelight

My favorite turn-on is:

- ❏ Kissing
- ❏ When you put your arms around me
- ❏ Nuzzling my neck
- ❏ None of the above, but I really like

_____

Music that gets me in the mood for lovemaking is:

- ❑ Our special song
- ❑ Classical
- ❑ Hot, steamy, with a pounding beat

My favorite place to make love is:

- ❑ The bedroom
- ❑ Somewhere else in the house:

  _____

- ❑ Outside/elsewhere: _____

When we make love, I prefer:

- ❑ You guiding my hands without words
- ❑ You letting me know what you want
- ❑ Leave it up to me . . . I'll decide

I love to make love most when:

- ❑ You're naked
- ❑ You let me undress you, and you undress me
- ❑ One (or both) of us still has some clothes on

My most precious memory of our lovemaking is:

_____

_____

_____

_____

_____

# Lube It or Lose It

Use a vaginal lubricant daily, not just prior to intercourse. Daily use of Astroglide, Slippery Stuff, or another lubricant can help restore moisture to dry tissue. "His and hers" lubricants are now available, so have some fun with these if you like. Warming lubricants are also available, but some women report that these products actually increase burning or irritation.

# Mess Around with the Way You Mess Around

The same old, same old makes anything boring—work, food, sex. If the time of day, position, and place where you have sex have become numbingly routine, change any of these, or all three. When you shift your timing, give thought not only to mid-morning or mid-afternoon instead of the customary evening coupling but also to slowing down the act. Sometimes when sex seems less comfortable and not quite as exciting in midlife, we may tend to rush through it. Slow down, breathe, and prolong the moment. Create a new space to make love and take a break from the bedroom. Use a spare room, a comfy couch or chair, the floor, stand up against the kitchen counters, or use the dining room table for something other than family meals—if it's sturdy enough, of course. Put a pillow or foam wedge under your hips to heighten your enjoyment. If you both prefer the bedroom, change the sheets, literally. Try a completely different color and texture—new silk, caressing flannel, or the softest cotton. Clear the room of books, papers, and any clutter so the emphasis in the room is on intimacy. A small bouquet of flowers; a candle with just the subtlest scent of sandalwood, rose, clove, or jasmine; and some fragrant massage oil can also be part of a room makeover that transforms a humdrum area into a heady love nest. And Shakespeare had it right when he said, "If music be the food of love, play on." Think about adding music as a background soundtrack to intimate moments—something that reminds you of your early courtship, a new artist, or lush classical sounds.

## Invest in Intimacy

Never bought a sex toy in your life? Are sensible flannels your customary bedroom attire? Think about investing in your intimate life with something new to wear or fun to play with. Consider a sexy nightie or a toy like the playfully named Pocket Rocket equally as important as staying current with fashion trends. After all, most of us don't think twice about updating our shoes or purses, and our love life merits the same attention.

## I Like to Watch

Research shows that women who report low sex drive in menopause still experience a rush of blood flow to the genitals when watching erotic films. This gust of sexual feeling can help boost your interest in having sex, so make a plan to watch your favorite sexy movie scene. Watch together before making love, or on your own if you prefer, to help you feel amorous the way you did in the old days. You may have your own favorite movies with sexy scenes, but here are some suggestions:

- *Body Heat*
- *The Bridges of Madison County*
- *Dirty Dancing*
- *From Here to Eternity*
- *Ghost*
- *The Notebook*
- *Notting Hill*
- *Out of Africa*
- *Rear Window*
- *Risky Business*
- *Something's Gotta Give*
- *Wild Things*

Here's something else to watch: your partner. Whether cuddling, massaging, or making love, do it with your eyes wide open. Look deeply and steadily into your beloved's eyes. This increased eye contact is a principle of Tantric lovemaking, where lovers achieve heightened intimacy by focusing more intensely on each other's eyes and breath, and the rest follows naturally.

# Think about It

Research shows that thinking about sex, and thinking about yourself as a highly sexual being, will increase your interest in having sex. Perhaps you've seen the cartoon jocularly depicting men's and women's brains, where most nooks and crannies in the man's brain are labeled *sex* (with the exception of a few designated *football* or *beer*), whereas women's brains are crammed with details about love, work, children, parents, birthdays, and anniversaries, with one tiny sex compartment.

Clichés aside, the detachment or indifference about sex that women experience in midlife can be replaced by a more mindful approach to the sensual and sexual part of our lives. What does this mean in a practical sense? Start by telling yourself regularly, "I am sexy." If you have felt shut off from the sexual excitement you once experienced, focus your mind actively on how your most memorable sexual encounters affected all five of your senses—touch, smell, taste, sound, sight. You can relive these moments whenever and wherever you choose, and cast your mind back to whom and what you touched, smelled, heard, saw, and tasted.

# Explore Other Ways to Be Intimate

Trade back, foot, or hand massages with your mate. Wrap up in each other's arms and watch something funny on TV. Read a poem out loud. Feed each other bites of something delicious. Get in the hot tub or shower together. Let your partner know that you want to be sensuous, and remember that not every erotic encounter has to include traditional intercourse. Be nude together somewhere other than the shower or bedroom if you live in a place that allows you that privacy. Never mind if your partner says he'd rather not sit down to lunch or read in the living room while nude— you can do it anyway. You'll be surprised by how good, and how free, it feels. Even if you partner doesn't join you, he'll notice, and chances are your experiment with new behavior will seem seductive and sensual to both of you.

## Exercise and Sex

Fatigue plagues many women in menopause and is frequently cited as the reason they crave sleep more than sex. Regular exercise not only boosts your energy and combats fatigue but can also provide a way to spend enjoyable time with your spouse. Some studies find that exercise increases testosterone, the hormone of desire, in women and men. Make a standing date to take a walk together after dinner without smartphones and strictly forbidding the topics of kids, money, and in-laws in conversation. Take a bike ride together on a weekend afternoon. Try a gentle yoga class specifically for couples. Along with producing a rise in testosterone, this form of exercise increases blood flow to the genital area. Or join a dance class for adults, where even a spouse who normally cringes on the dance floor can relax and enjoy the music and gentle coaching on dance steps. Then see what happens when you put on some music before making love. Dance by yourself if you like, wearing something soft and sexy—or dance wearing nothing at all.

## Spice It Up

The notion of certain foods as aphrodisiacs goes back thousands of years. The science documenting any measurable increase in sex drive or performance after eating certain foods is sketchy, although a recent study in the *International Food Research Journal* showed that saffron and ginseng may cause blood to pulse more effectively, possibly boosting sexual performance. However, it's indisputable that a romantic meal of colorful, delicious, and possibly aphrodisiacal dishes is a pleasurable and sensuous experience. Rather than limiting special meals to birthdays or anniversaries, make a habit of them. Plan, shop for, and prepare the meal together, listening to music while you cook. Or put a picnic together and take it to a beach, lake, or park when the weather allows. Include tasty, healthy foods like arugula, pine nuts, raspberries, saffron rice, salmon with fennel, pineapple, oysters, fresh figs, asparagus—all believed to increase amorous feelings—and don't forget a sip of red wine and a bite of dark chocolate for dessert.

## Do It Yourself

Some experts recommend more frequent intercourse to increase lubrication and to gradually and gently stretch a narrowed vaginal opening. Self-stimulation—where you control the what, where, when, and how much—is another way to help make sex more comfortable so you can enjoy it more with a partner. Vaginal dilators or vibrators can help. A group of women ranging in age from their forties to their sixties roared laughing recently when one of them reported finding a *Twilight* vaginal dilator that was white, with sparkles, on the Internet. She didn't cop to buying it, but everyone got the idea.

Sensual pleasure may evolve in midlife, and if you've had a lull in desire or interest, don't worry too much. The doldrums won't be permanent after you've tried some of today's tips. You'll find that freedom to explore different ways of experiencing sexual satisfaction can bring more enjoyment, not less.

DAY 6

# MUNCHIES

Today is the day you'll start to recalibrate what you eat so you can enjoy healthy, colorful, easy-to-prepare food without going up a pants size. Menopause marks the time when our metabolism can shift into a sluggish mode, meaning that even when eating less, many women find their shape growing softer and rounder. Less testosterone can cause muscles to slacken and lose tone, so even if the number on the scale hasn't changed much, your weight is distributed differently and you may look and feel heavier.

Menopause can also be a time of odd cravings—one woman told of existing on a none-too-nutritious mix of orange peanut butter crackers often found in vending machines, circus peanut candy, and Vienna Fingers. Another described subsisting on potatoes and bread—she couldn't seem to get enough carbohydrates.

On the other hand, some women experience loss of appetite in menopause. This can be tied in with depression or a feeling of being bored and burdened by the grind of food shopping, getting the meals on the table, and cleaning up afterward. Other women, newly alone because they are divorced or widowed or their children have left home, feel like they can't be bothered with food. And some women find the foods they once enjoyed now trigger bouts of heartburn. Smooth muscle tissue that propels food through the digestive tract also changes as a result of dwindling estrogen and testosterone, which is why some women report more indigestion and heartburn during menopause.

If any of these scenarios holds true for you, today is the day you'll reverse that pattern. You'll adopt a new equation that lets you eat more and weigh less simply by savoring the foods that pack the most nutritional power. Food is medicine during menopause, and you're eating to feed body and soul. Limiting certain foods, adding new combinations, and timing meals and snacks can help manage hot flashes, insomnia, fatigue, and anxiety and can help avoid heartburn. Eating more healthy, colorful foods also means that you don't have to feel hungry or worry that every bite ends up showing on your hips or thighs. Your appetite for an enjoyment of good foods can enliven your skin and hair as well.

# Battle Stress and Fatigue with Breakfast

Research shows that if you pile on the protein at breakfast, you'll reduce your food cravings later in the day and resist overeating. MRI brain images of people who had eaten a high-protein breakfast revealed less activity in the portion of the brain that controls food motivation and reward. That translates into less desire to grab a muffin, chips, or M&Ms to stave off hunger later in the day. In addition, starting your day with a healthy breakfast lets you ward off those dips in blood sugar levels that can produce an edgy, tearful feeling. Steady blood sugar levels also help keep your adrenal glands from spiking your cortisol levels. Cortisol is the stress hormone that dampens immune response when produced in excess.

Now, piling on the protein doesn't mean sitting down to an NFL-style repast with a dozen eggs and a pound of bacon, of course. Simple, quick, and delicious ways to include protein in your breakfast include

- Yogurt and a mix of bright red and blue berries—choose Greek-style yogurt for more protein and calcium.

- A sliver of smoked salmon with cream cheese on a whole-grain bagel.

- Granola or oatmeal topped with sliced banana and a dash of wheat germ for extra protein. If the word *germ* or visions of unkempt hippies have kept you away from this protein powerhouse, give it a try! It's nutty and delicious. Shake on the cinnamon too. Everything nice about this fragrant spice includes its potential to inhibit growth of toxic amyloid fibrils, which make up the plaque found with Alzheimer's disease. Cinnamon is also linked to improved glucose, insulin, cholesterol, and HbA1c levels in people with type 2 diabetes.

- An appetizer of string cheese and whole-grain crackers, and a breakfast cocktail of 100 percent grape juice. Why wait until five p.m. for happy hour? Research suggests that the flavonoids and resveratrol in grape juice can help steady your blood pressure and keep your LDL, or bad cholesterol, low.

- Two scrambled eggs wrapped in a warm tortilla—topped with salsa for a kick if you like. Salsa contains lycopene, an antioxidant that may reduce cancer risk, according to observational studies of people who ate a diet high in lycopene from tomato-based foods like salsa and tomato sauce. Sometimes spicy foods can set off hot flashes, but choosing a mild salsa can avoid that.

- Café au lait made with lots of hot, low-fat milk and multigrain toast topped with almond or cashew butter. Plain old peanut butter is fine too.

- A smoothie made with fresh or frozen berries, banana, yogurt, and a splash of 100 percent juice—especially tasty on a muggy summer morning.

- Two hard-boiled eggs, a crispy apple or juicy orange, low-fat milk, and a handful of trail mix will do when you're pressed for time. Hard-boil a few eggs ahead of time and keep them in the fridge to grab on the go. If you're concerned about cholesterol, eat just the hard-boiled egg white—it's a perfect protein but contains no cholesterol.

Many women say, "I don't have time for breakfast," or "I never feel like eating breakfast." If you fall into that category, reconsider breakfast as a way of slowing down and taking care of yourself. The few minutes you set aside to nourish yourself in the morning are an investment in having a better day. Use a pretty, favorite cup or plate and try to avoid the television or the smartphone while you eat. Give yourself this brief time to center and quiet your spirit, preparing to enjoy the day.

## Lunch for Lasting Health

During menopause, we all need to become ladies who lunch—not necessarily with tablecloths, silver, and crystal in a fine restaurant, although wouldn't that be nice? Today you're going to start paying more attention to your lunch, which is a way of paying attention to yourself. Lunch isn't a luxury, nor is it something to cram absently into your mouth while you're doing something else. Your lunch needs to fuel your energy, strengthen your bones, calm your nerves, and boost your heart health. And you can do this every day with just a little planning.

What is your current style of eating lunch?

- ❏ I usually skip lunch.
- ❏ I don't think about lunch until I'm starving, and then I often grab something from the drive-through or vending machine.

❑ I eat lunch quickly at my desk so I can keep working.

❑ I eat a healthy lunch almost every day.

If you usually skip or cram your lunch, today is the day to slow down and start enjoying a healthy midday break. If you checked the last box, good for you, but read on anyway to learn how to add spice and color to your lunches and to increase their healthy impact every day.

Who said lunch has to be routine or dull? Here are some suggestions to help you climb out of your lunch rut.

## Make a New Salad

Toss arugula, also known as rocket, with olive oil, lemon, and a bit of salt. This bright, easy salad packs in vitamins A, C, and K and ups your calcium intake too. Shave on an ounce of Parmesan cheese to add 10 grams of protein and enjoy with crispy whole-grain crackers or chewy bread.

## Try Wraps Instead of Sandwiches

Fold a tomato or spinach wrap around chopped salad with feta or blue cheese, or around lean turkey or chicken. Make a delicious Asian-style wrap with canned salmon tossed with chopped scallions, chopped cucumber, and some left-over rice tossed with sesame-ginger vinaigrette. Add shredded veggies—carrots, lettuce, or broccoli slaw—to any wrap for extra crunch and vitamins. You can make these wraps from scratch if you have time, or you can buy prepared salad greens and chopped veggies from the salad bar at the grocery to speed the process. If you think the salad bar is too pricey, consider that you will be more likely to eat the food before it wilts or browns when you don't have to be the one to chop it. You'll waste less and eat better. You're worth any extra cost, and your lunch will be tasty, colorful, and nutritious.

## Spice Up Your Lunch with Turmeric

Turmeric is a deep orange-yellow spice that has been considered both medicine and food for centuries due to its anti-inflammatory properties. Devil a couple of eggs with turmeric mixed with a bit of mayo, and toss in some snipped chives or finely diced scallions. Or put a dash of turmeric in egg salad or tuna salad. You'll give your lunch a rich hue and a nutritional boost.

## Use Cayenne for Energy and to Curb Appetite

Researchers at Purdue University found that capsaicin, the compound in cayenne pepper, cuts appetite and increases energy. Shake a bit of ground cayenne pepper or dried red pepper flakes on a salad, fruit cup, or cottage cheese. This natural appetite suppressant appears to affect the portion of the brain that controls food motivation and reward, so a taste of it at lunch may keep you from craving candy at three p.m. This spice packs a punch, though, so use it sparingly.

# Swap Out the Apple, Banana, or Orange

Apples, bananas, and oranges are nutritious and delicious standby fruits, but think about adding new fruits to your lunch to break up the routine. Squeeze lime over seasonal melon or mango, or enjoy fresh pineapple chunks that are loaded with vitamin C and fiber. Pineapple may also help ease heartburn, which plagues many women in menopause. Its sweetness can also satisfy cravings for less healthy sugary foods.

Savor the beautiful ruby color and tangy taste of pomegranate. This ancient fruit is loaded with disease-fighting antioxidants. Not sure how to eat a pomegranate? Score it into six sections, and then cut off the top. Pull the sections apart gently, and use your thumbs to turn them out. Carefully remove the delicious, jewel-like seeds. This isn't nearly as hard or time-consuming as you might think, and the health rewards of this delectable fruit are well worth it.

# Have Dessert!

You may decide to have your daily medicinal dose of dark chocolate at lunch or to enjoy a couple of zesty gingersnaps, delicate wafers, or other cookies for a small treat. Indulging in a modest dessert at midday boosts your mood—or your memory if you choose a bit of dark chocolate—and helps make lunch a pleasant ritual rather than a rushed affair.

# Dine to Fall Asleep

Well, don't fall asleep at the table, exactly, but think about how your dinner can double as your sleep aid. The type and amount of food you choose can help promote more restful nights. Add foods that are high in the amino acid tryptophan to your evening meal. These include turkey, tuna, bananas, dates, figs, and milk. The quickest and easiest way to do this is to enjoy a glass of low-fat milk with your dinner, but if that's not to your taste, you can stir low-fat milk into soups or Alfredo sauce for pasta or vegetables. Or make comforting macaroni and cheese with low-fat milk, reduced-fat cheese or light cream cheese, whole-grain pasta if you like it, and a tablespoon of butter.

You can also stir pureed vegetables into your macaroni and cheese or other pasta dishes. Use pureed cauliflower, carrots, or winter squash (a great source of omega-3 fatty acids). A study in *The American Journal of Clinical Nutrition* demonstrated that adding extra pureed vegetables to certain dishes meant that study participants ate 200 to 350 fewer calories and did not notice a taste difference. The extra veggies fill you up and increase the nutritional punch of the dish. You can also add spinach or sun-dried tomatoes for extra vitamin C, vitamin K, and iron.

Stumped on how to get figs or dates into dinner? Snip dried figs and add them to your favorite stew recipe made with lean beef, vegetables, and lentils. The figs add fiber, potassium, sleep-promoting tryptophan, and a rich nutty flavor to the dish. The next time you roast chicken in the oven, line the baking dish with lemon slices and dried figs. Before you put the dish in the oven, sprinkle the chicken, lemon, and figs with a bit of brown sugar and salt and drizzle with lemon juice. The fruit will roast with the chicken, look beautiful on the plate, and pack more nutrients into your dinner.

Your salad will be terrific—and soporific—if you sprinkle on a few chopped dates. Or stir chopped dates along with toasted almonds into a side dish of couscous. Dates are always a delicious addition to fruit salad for dessert too.

Keep your dinner on the light side—and not too sweet—to help you sleep too. A heavy meal sitting in your stomach can interrupt your rest. Too much sugar can bring on the jitters and make it harder for you to wind down in the evening.

# Snack on Vitamin $B_{12}$, Vitamin D, and Omega-3s

Chances are that if you're like most women in midlife, you are probably not getting enough of these three key nutrients every day: omega-3s, vitamin D, and vitamin $B_{12}$. In fact, a shortage of $B_{12}$ is often overlooked when women describe fatigue, a racing heart, or foggy memory. You need 2.4 micrograms (mcg) of $B_{12}$ daily for red blood cell formation and sharp cognitive function.

A vitamin D deficiency produces weak muscles and porous, brittle bones, and it spikes your risk for heart disease, certain cancers, and diabetes. Aim for 600 international units (IU) daily. Vitamin D helps your body absorb calcium, which is especially important during menopause when estrogen decline plays a significant role in bone loss.

Omega-3 fatty acids reduce your risk for cardiovascular disease, abnormal heartbeats, high triglycerides, and clogged arteries. There is no recommended daily amount of this nutrient, but the American Heart Association suggests that eating two small servings, about 3.5 ounces, of fatty fish per week can help you get an adequate amount in your diet. Walnuts and flaxseed are also excellent sources of omega-3s.

When you're hungry at mid-morning, mid-afternoon, or in the evening, by all means, reach for fruits and veggies for their vitamins, minerals, and fiber. Rather than starving yourself, consider snacks or mini-meals as part of a solid nutritional plan. And snack time is your chance to supplement your omega-3, vitamin D, and vitamin $B_{12}$ intake. Vary your snack schedule with a nosh from the list below. These foods provide some of the three nutrients often missing from our diets. You'll stave off your hunger at the same time you keep your heart, bones, and muscles strong, your memory keen, and your energy steady.

- Whole-grain cereal fortified with vitamin $B_{12}$ and low-fat milk. Keep a small resealable bag of the cereal in your purse or car—you can munch on it as a snack even if you don't have milk handy. Sprinkle on ground flaxseed for an extra boost.

- Walnuts. Enjoy them plain or candy them for an occasional treat. Most recipes for candied walnuts call for a half cup or more of sugar for a pound of walnuts. You can easily cut that in half. Beat 1 egg white and add 2 tablespoons cinnamon, 1 tablespoon vanilla, ¼ cup sugar, and coat the nuts. Line a cookie sheet with parchment paper, and spread the nuts on it. Roast at 300°F for 30 minutes. Divvy them into plenty of small snack bags that you can keep on hand in your purse or glove compartment.

- Hard-boiled egg. Prepare as many as you like in advance and keep them in the fridge for quick snacks. Sprinkle on some Cajun seasoning for color and kick, or just plain paprika if you like a milder flavor. Or slice the hard-boiled egg in half and add just the tiniest dab of mayo to each half. They're like quick deviled eggs, without the fuss and with a fraction of the fat and calories.

- Half tuna sandwich. Add shredded carrot or chopped onion or cucumber for a vegetable nutrient boost. Tuck the tuna into half a pita or make it on dark, chewy pumpernickel for a change.

- Anchovies. Are you raising your eyebrows, wondering how you're going to snack on anchovies at your desk? Or are you protesting, "I don't *like* anchovies." But you can make an appetizing dip with 4 anchovies, olive oil, 3 roasted peppers, and 3 or 4 cloves of roasted garlic. Whirl it all in the blender with just enough olive oil to make a smooth dip. This is delicious served with vegetables or chunks of bread. Anchovies pack a lot of salt, but they are also a great source of omega-3s and calcium too.

END YOUR MENOPAUSE MISERY

## Water Things Down

Sip water throughout the day to keep your energy up and to hydrate your hair, skin, and nails. Lack of fluid can worsen the fatigue that so many women experience in menopause. Adding slices of lemon or cucumber to your water has a mildly diuretic effect and can also help avoid that bloated or puffy feeling. If you have a tendency to pop open a can of diet soda for a jolt of caffeine or to fill you up temporarily, try weaning yourself off. Cut back on the amount of soda you down daily, and drink an equal amount of water. Women who drink three or more cola sodas per day have significantly lower bone density. Researchers aren't sure whether the caffeine and phosphorus in cola are to blame or whether the cola-drinking group drinks less milk and therefore consumes less calcium. A study in *The Journal of General Internal Medicine* showed that daily diet soda drinkers had an elevated risk of heart attack and stroke when compared with people who drank regular soda or who drank diet soda less often than daily. An occasional soda, diet or regular, is fine, but rely on water as your primary source of hydration.

## Mix Calcium into Your Menu in Menopause

After age fifty-one, we need 1,200 milligrams (mg) of calcium daily to protect against bone loss. You can get enough of this mighty mineral with two to four servings of calcium-rich foods a day. Dairy sources include low-fat milk, yogurt, and cheese, but some women just aren't big milk drinkers or cheese or yogurt eaters. That's okay—you can also get bone-strengthening calcium from nondairy choices like soy milk, broccoli, and leafy green vegetables such as collard greens and mustard greens.

Made with bacon or ham, greens are a Southern staple, but you can make an equally tasty but healthier version by plunging the greens into lightly salted boiling water and cooking until tender. Drain the greens, press out the moisture, and then toss them into a skillet where you have heated some olive oil and garlic. Stir quickly, just until coated and heated through, and serve with lemon or vinegar for a side dish that sustains your bones. Baby bok choy makes a scrumptious salad if you chop it; add sliced green onions and toasted almond slivers; and drizzle with a dressing made with oil, vinegar, a dash of sugar, and a splash of soy sauce. Bottled Asian-style dressing also works well with this crispy, flavorful salad. For extra fun and crunch, top with a sprinkling of chow mein noodles.

And because adding a touch of sweetness to life is always a good thing, remember that molasses is an excellent source of calcium too. A tablespoon of blackstrap molasses delivers 137 mg of calcium. Stir some molasses into your coffee or drizzle it on hot cereal. If you like to bake, consider your gingerbread or molasses cookie recipe part of your bone-healthy diet—molasses gives these treats a rich flavor and a calcium boost.

# Food Values

More than just sustenance, food reflects the way in which we value ourselves. Ignoring food until we are starving and then eating any old thing really is a way of ignoring ourselves. Or stuffing food furtively, absently, or nervously often represents an effort to quell feelings of anxiety or discontent. As you think about your food today, try at least one of the suggestions you've just read about, and enjoy the healthy, colorful foods that look pretty on your plate and add to your good health. In menopause, your nourishment becomes more important than ever in staying strong, satisfied, and serene.

# Keeping Healthy Company

As important as what we eat during the perimenopausal transition is, when we eat and with whom count too. Just as your soothing cup of tea can prevent the buildup of harmful plaque in the arteries and your leafy green vegetables build bones, your ongoing social activities have health benefits too. Schedule a regular get-together with friends for tea. Make a priority of having a monthly lunch where you and friends discuss a book or perhaps quilt or knit together. In people of all ages, the camaraderie of a standing dinner date can help lower heart disease risk and reduce the likelihood of depression too. Regular and strong social support is linked to dampened stress levels, lower blood pressure, and a more robust immune response. Sharing love, laughter, and good food with friends and family is part of your healthy routine in menopause.

# MUSCLE AND BONE

Today let's hone in on what you can do to keep your muscles toned—including the most important muscle of all: your heart—and keep your bones in good shape. If just the word *exercise* makes you feel like you want to lie down, don't worry. You'll learn ways to get going gently with regular activity to avert the blues, boost your alertness, and promote sound sleep.

The connection between muscle and brain becomes even more critical during menopause than it has been your entire life. Study after study shows that mature adults who are active not only live longer with lower incidence of chronic illnesses such as heart disease and diabetes, but they also report greater satisfaction with life and less depression. If exercise were a pill or a potion, it would be hawked as a powerful health solution, but it doesn't have to cost a cent. It provides longevity, a brighter mood, more restful sleep, and possibly even a revved-up sex drive. Regular activity today reduces your likelihood of a heart attack or dependence on a walker tomorrow. With claims like these, we'd probably all rush out to get whatever it was that could deliver these robust benefits. It's always available, yet many of us let boredom or inertia get in the way of exercising, or we claim that we can't find the time.

Which statement most closely reflects how you feel about exercise?

- ❑ I exercise only sporadically. I'll stick with an exercise program for a while, but then I slack off.
- ❑ I'd like to be more active, but finding the time to exercise always poses a challenge for me.
- ❑ Exercise is a burden and a bore, and I hardly ever do it.
- ❑ I spend time thinking that I should exercise and then feel guilty because I don't.
- ❑ I used to get more exercise, but lately I find that motivating myself gets harder and I tend to put off exercising more than I used to.
- ❑ I try to get thirty minutes of exercise on most days of the week.
- ❑ I force myself to exercise, but I don't enjoy it and I spend the entire time wanting it to be over.
- ❑ I've been doing the same kind of exercise for a long time, and I am bored with it now, but I don't feel motivated to make a change.

You probably know all this, but just in case you need a bit of a refresher, there are several reasons why you'll want to make regular exercise part of your routine, as essential as eating, sleeping, drinking water, and bathing.

Although we tend to worry more about breast cancer than other diseases, heart disease causes more deaths in women every year than breast, ovarian, and lung cancer combined. One in four women dies from heart disease, according to the National Heart, Lung, and Blood Institute. Estrogen has a protective effect on the heart, and the loss of this effect ups the risk for heart disease. Exercise offers a simple and achievable way to help counteract this risk. In a study of twenty-seven thousand women who took part in the Women's Health Study, researchers analyzed heart disease risk factors and exercise levels. They found a 40 percent reduction in heart attack and stroke between the highest and lowest exercise groups. The highest exercise group took part in five or more hours of moderate-intensity exercise, such as brisk walking, per week. The lowest exercise group had less than one hour of physical activity per week.

Thinning, fragile bones from osteoporosis affect four times as many women as men, increasing the risk for fracture. Bone loss can cause women to shrink during the menopausal years, giving a new, unwelcome meaning to the phrase *little old lady*. Keeping active today keeps your bones strong and lowers the risk of fracture in the future. The American Academy of Orthopedic Surgeons reports that most people who suffer a hip fracture do not live independently afterward. They either require assistance at home or, in 40 percent of hip fracture cases in people older than sixty-five, they must move to a long-term care facility (that's pleasant speak for a nursing home, of course). A hip fracture means using a cane or walker for several months after the injury, and in nearly half of these cases, the cane or walker becomes a permanent requirement. And here is an even more alarming statistic: about 24 percent of people who suffer a hip fracture when they are older than fifty die within twelve months due to complications related to the injury and the extended recovery period. Yes, a hip fracture, walker, and nursing home may seem like a remote possibility today, but to keep it that way and not let it turn into a debilitating reality, we need gentle daily exercise.

Exercise also helps you slim your hips and build up your hippocampus. It builds lean muscle, which burns more calories than fat. Even moderate exercise boosts your metabolism, helps your clothes fit better, spikes your energy and alertness, and helps ward off bouts of teariness or anxiety. Another exercise bonus: it increases the size of your hippocampus, the brain structure that is essential to memory formation. A study of older adults with dementia found that walking forty minutes a day, three times a week, resulted in a measurable increase in hippocampus size as well as improved performance on memory tests.

Ease joint pain by exercising. Many women complain of feeling creaky during menopause, with joint aches and pains that never seemed to be there before. Falling estrogen levels and the loss of its anti-inflammatory effects are implicated in this change-of-life creakiness, but many women worry it signals arthritis. Although it may seem counterintuitive to move around when you're feeling achy, you'll find that exercise actually helps relieve joint pain. This occurs in two ways. First, as you strengthen the muscles that surround your joints, you take pressure off them. Weaker muscles mean more pressure on joints, and more discomfort. Second, trimming even one pound from your weight takes four pounds of pressure off your knees, according to Wake Forest University researchers. They didn't measure how much each pound of weight loss reduced pressure on ankle or hip joints, but it stands to reason that the same principle would apply.

Exercise means better rest. If you're exercising at night in bed by tossing and turning, try moving around more during the day to smooth out your sleep patterns. As part of the National Health and Nutrition Examination Survey, researchers analyzed a representative sample of more than 2,600 adults of all ages. Just over twenty minutes of exercise a day, or 150 minutes a week, was associated with a 65 percent improvement in sleep quality and less daytime sleepiness. Maybe you're caught in that nasty cycle of feeling too fatigued to exercise because you sleep so poorly at night. Today is the day you can begin to reverse that trend, even if you start with just ten minutes of walking.

Lift your mood. Your brain rewards you for your exercise efforts, big and small, by releasing endorphins, the body's natural pain relievers. The endorphin payoff also includes a feel-good sensation, appetite modulation, release of sex hormones, and a boost in your immune response. People who experience anxiety or panic disorders reduce their stress response when they stay active. And here's more good news: the latest science on exercise and depression shows that even light activity helps. In a population study of more than forty thousand people, Norwegian researchers found that light activity—defined as any activity not leading to being sweaty or out of breath—was associated with significantly fewer depressive symptoms. Lots of women really like the part about not getting sweaty. Try a ten-minute morning walk—you'll up your heart rate and metabolism, increase your blood flow and energy, and feel more positive and alert.

What's more, recurrent depression and stress shorten the telomere, the outer part of a chromosome. The length of the telomere is linked with age-related diseases. Exercise that helps keep depression at bay helps you live not only better but also longer. So the next time you're tempted to put off that ten-minute walk, convince yourself to get out there and lengthen your telomere!

## Try It, You'll Like It

Did your mother have a copy of *The I Hate to Cook Book* by Peg Bracken, the witty recipe collection published in 1960, that instructed women to "stare sullenly at the sink" while they concocted dinner with noodles and bouillon cubes? If you feel like you could be a modern-day author of *The I Hate to Exercise Book* or if just the thought of exercising makes you want to lie down, try these simple, easy, and fun tips. They'll help you get started if you haven't exercised recently, and they'll give you ideas on changing up your routine if you're tired of the same old, same old.

## Dress Up

No aging or stained sweats or T-shirts allowed. Comfortable exercise wear comes in smart-looking designs and colors so you can look and feel good. Invest in an exercise outfit that doubles as casual wear and lets you easily stop at the market or run any errand on your way to or from being active.

## Buddy Up

Enlist a friend, sister, cousin, coworker, or neighbor to take a regular walk, and make a standing date. Knowing that someone is counting on you makes it harder to put off exercising. And don't forget about the support you can get from a nonhuman exercise buddy. If you have a dog, add an extra walk—your pet will love you for it. No dog and don't want to adopt one? You may have neighbors who wouldn't mind at all if you took their pup for an extra stroll.

## Change It Up

Vary your routine to move different sets of muscles and to ward off tedium. If you're just starting out with exercise and walking suits you best, choose different routes on different days of the week. You'll see new people and take in another view of the landscape. For hints on varying the scenery, take a look at *www.traillink.com,* which shows walking and biking trails with a full description of their length and level of ease or difficulty. You may be surprised to find hidden and beautiful areas very near you. And if you have an exercise routine in place but you're tired of it, add variety either by switching the order in which you do the exercises, joining a different group or class, or incorporating a fresh form of activity.

## Learn Something New While You Keep Fit

Dancing is terrific exercise, and many communities offer reasonably priced dance lessons and classes through the recreation department. Try a dancing style you've never attempted—the music will energize you and you'll find that it's impossible to feel stressed or worried while you're dancing. Or take a tennis or golf lesson to gain a new skill that helps keep you mentally sharp and physically fit at the same time. A fitness drumming class is another way to get a great workout, and you can imagine yourself pounding on anything (or anyone) you like. If you favor quieter, more slow-paced activity, consider a tai chi or qi gong class, both of which take you through deep breathing and slow, measured movements with a calm sense of strength and control. Trying a new activity also offers the bonuses of a boost in energy and increased social contact, which can help avoid depression and anxiety.

## Be an Exercise Homebody If You Like

No law says you have to go *out* and exercise every day. Whether rain, biting cold, or muggy heat make you want to stay indoors, or if you simply enjoy being at home, keep active while you're there. Stand up and balance on one foot while you talk on the phone, turn on the music and dance, take the stairs at a brisk clip, grab a fifteen-ounce can from the cupboard and hoist it as a no-cost weight system. Tone your biceps while you watch television by holding the can and raising your arms above your shoulders or by doing curls, where you lift the can from your waist to your shoulder. Household chores count as exercise too. Organizing a closet, scrubbing a floor, and washing a car aren't at the top of anyone's list of fun things to do, but these tasks rev up your metabolism, clear your mind, and give you the satisfaction of accomplishing a job while keeping yourself strong.

## Make Exercise a Hobby

Did you know that you burn approximately 167 calories in a half hour when you're gardening? When you dig, weed, rake, plant seedlings, and harvest, you're keeping your heart, bones, and muscles strong too. Stephanie's grandparents were Michigan farmers whose daily lives included all these activities. They lived robust, healthy lives until they were ninety and ninety-seven! Gardening in the sun also allows your skin to produce vitamin D, which helps protect against weak muscles, brittle bones, heart disease, certain cancers, and diabetes. Vitamin D also improves your uptake of calcium, which is especially important in menopause. Moderate your sun exposure to guard against skin cancer—wear a wide-brimmed hat and sunscreen with an SPF of 15 or higher while you get out and dig, and try to garden before ten a.m. or after two p.m. No yard? A sunny spot on your porch, patio, or doorstep will do to grow your own crops in containers. Tomatoes, peppers, eggplants, green onions, beans, lettuce, squash, radishes, and parsley will thrive in containers. You'll not only join the demographic of gardeners older than fifty who reported high life satisfaction in a research study, but you'll be more likely to eat extra veggies too.

## Everybody in the Pool

When you go for a dip, swimming is not only easy on your body, but it also uses all your muscle groups: legs, abs, shoulders, back, glutes, and hips. The water's resistance helps you build strength quickly, even if you decide to start by swimming only a lap or two at a time, or just walking in the pool. Many gyms or community recreation programs offer water exercise classes, which can be a fun way to socialize and increase your strength at the same time. Swimming can also be meditative and relaxing—the sound and feel of the water can help to quiet and focus the mind.

## Relive Your Youth with Exercise

If you tend to want to say, "Not it!" when you think about exercise, try an activity you enjoyed as a child but perhaps haven't done in years. Hop on a bike, spin a hula hoop, or get out a jump rope and sift through your memory for as many of those schoolyard chants as you can recollect. "Oh, Mary

Mack Mack Mack, all dressed in black black black . . ." Did you skate when you were a girl? Check out an ice- or roller-skating arena in your community to see if adult sessions are offered. And remember that playing counts as exercise too. If you're a grandmother, your grandchildren will be delighted to launch a game of tag, hide-and-seek, or even the simple chase-me game that toddlers adore.

## Have an Adventure

Exercise doesn't have to mean a numbingly dull walk to nowhere on a treadmill. Recruit a plucky friend to occasionally try something different that combines a workout and a new experience. Take a kayak or canoe out on a lake or the ocean if it's nearby, or sign up for a sailing lesson. Try an afternoon of horseback riding for a complete change of routine. If there is a rock-climbing gym in your town that offers a fun and safe way to scale new heights, try it. Find a women's boxing or other martial arts class to increase your fitness and your sense of personal safety. Brandish a sword and declare, "*En garde!*" at a fencing lesson. Any of these, even as an occasional adventure or exercise bonus, can combine benefits to your muscles and bones with the mental exhilaration of taking on a new challenge and learning something fresh.

## Fulfill Other Needs with Exercise

Sometimes it helps to think about exercise as meeting other needs in your life besides the activity itself. For instance, if you love music but find that you rarely have time to listen to it anymore, listen while you exercise. Or if you feel that your days are filled with nonstop demands from others, consider a walk as precious time for yourself, a form of moving meditation. Connecting exercise to something else that is important helps us to stay motivated.

## Just One Dance

If you're still feeling like exercise just isn't your thing, try this: put on just one fast song that you love and dance to it in the privacy of your home. You'll bump your heart rate and give yourself the awareness, for just a moment, of how good it can feel. That may prompt you to do it again.

You'll do your body and your spirit a favor when you try some of these tips on staying active. Keep an open mind and remember that you don't have to sign on to any one of these activities forever. Try one activity one week and see how you like it. Reward your exercise effort at least once a month with flowers, a new book, a movie, a pedicure—something that reinforces the good feelings you get from exercise. Experiment, have fun, seek company, and we guarantee you'll like the way you look and feel.

# MOISTURE

The term *leaky vessel* can take on new and unwelcome meaning in menopause, particularly on days when it feels as if our bodies are betraying us by sweating and leaking at the most inopportune times. Escalating dry-cleaning bills and outsized loads of laundry are a real, but less discussed, aspect of the menopausal transition. If your body has been behaving unpredictably, with rushes of heat to your face and torso in the middle of the day or rivulets of sweat by night, take heart. Today, you'll find out how to tame hot flashes. With a few easy-to-master tips and exercises, you can trade the discomfort, inconvenience, interrupted sleep, and time spent changing and washing clothing and bedding for other things you like to do. If urine leaks out with every laugh, cough, or sneeze, today you'll begin strengthening your pelvic muscles so you don't need to spend as much time or energy scoping out the nearest ladies' room at any destination.

## The Thermostat Is Off

No one understands the exact mechanism behind hot flashes. One theory is that your body's waning production of estrogen interferes with the function of the hypothalamus, the area at the base of your brain that regulates temperature. Your body heat doesn't actually spike, but your brain responds as if it did, so the blood vessels underneath your skin dilate in order to cool you down. Flushing, sweating, skin redness or blotchiness, and sometimes rapid heartbeat can occur with a hot flash. After a hot flash, you may suddenly feel like you're freezing as your body attempts to get the temperature signals straight.

Hot flashes are as varied as the women they affect. Some data suggests that 40 percent of women experience hot flashes, while other estimates go as high as 80 percent. Some women have hot flashes only occasionally, and others have them many times a day and throughout the night. They can last for a few seconds or several minutes. Some women say they can tell when a hot flash is coming on because their skin begins to tingle, while others describe the surge of heat and sweat that comes with no warning. Many women report hot flashes that seem to travel from the waist or chest up to the neck, face, and scalp, with sweating that breaks out on these parts of the body as the sensation of heat rushes upward.

It may be slim comfort, but recent research revealed that hot flashes are linked with a lower incidence of cardiovascular disease. While hot flashes and night sweats were once believed to be part of vascular problems occurring when women's hormone levels decline, a review of medical information from sixty thousand women who took part in the Women's Health Initiative Observational Study showed that women who had hot flashes early in menopause had fewer cardiovascular events than women who had them late in menopause or not at all. The observational study tracked women ages fifty to seventy-nine for an average of eight years. More research may reveal that hot flashes and night sweats are the body's way of boosting circulation to counteract an estrogen-related slow in blood flow. Let's look at other ways to keep your circulation steady that don't require mopping your brow or changing your sheets.

## Eat to Stay Cool

What you had for lunch could have triggered that afternoon outbreak of sweat, just as your dinner can be related to that damp one a.m. wakeup. Hot foods and spices, as well as alcohol, are notorious for bringing on a rush of heat and sweating in menopausal women. The stimulating effect of caffeine prompts hot flashes, as can too much sugar, possibly related to the swing in blood sugar levels. You don't have to give up spicy food for bland pabulum, but there are a few things you should know to help you manage food-related hot flashes or night sweats.

- If you love foods with chili, cayenne, or curry, reduce the amount of these spices in the recipe when you cook.

- When you enjoy spicy foods in Thai, Mexican, Indian, or other restaurants, eat a smaller portion of the spicy dish and balance it with a cooling green salad with cucumbers and radishes, or a fruit salad with strawberries and watermelon sprinkled with chopped fresh mint.

- Wait until your food cools a bit before you eat it. Hot flashes are triggered not only by the heat of spices, but food that is very hot in temperature can also make you break a sweat.

- If coffee or tea is a morning must for you, see if limiting your wakeup beverage to one cup per day helps cut hot flashes. And as with food, drinking your coffee or tea at just a slightly lower temperature can help too.

- Even one cocktail or one glass of wine can bring on a bout of flushing and sweating. You can shed a top layer before lifting your glass, or swap out that celebratory toast for sparkling water or juice.

## Look Cool While You Stay Cool

Layer your clothes so you can peel off a blouse or light jacket if you feel like you're hitting the boiling point. A camisole, shell, or T-shirt made of moisture-wicking fabric lets your skin breathe. Sporting goods or outdoor equipment stores are good places to look for these fabrics. The designers of these moisture-wicking pieces now make them in an array of colors and styles—gone are the days when this type of clothing was limited to serviceable-looking, dun-colored frumpiness. You can also select socks and underwear made from material that wicks moisture away from your skin. Stay away from cotton and polyester, which stay sodden after you've broken a sweat.

A light blouse over your shell or T-shirt gives you the option of shedding it if things heat up. In frostier weather, a jacket made from ultrathin, warm fabric can keep you from winter's chill without the bulk or weight that can be uncomfortable for women with hot flashes.

Remember to keep it loose, literally. Avoid clothing that constricts you anywhere, particularly around the waist. Choose pants and skirts with a supple waistband. While it may be tempting to don a turtleneck on a cold day, the fabric around your throat can feel like a vise if a hot flash comes on. Choose a blouse or shirt with a regular collar instead, and add a light wool or silk scarf for warmth. You can unwind the scarf easily if you feel yourself starting to flush. And if you've been wearing the same bra size for ages, now is a good time to have an experienced salesperson check your fit. You may need a different size or style of bra to help avoid feeling constrained and sweaty.

## Move to Stay Dry

Your exercise routine also goes a long way in helping you to control hot flashes and night sweats. "But wait," you might say. "How does getting sweaty from exercise help me to stop sweating?" Exercise may diminish the surges of follicle stimulating hormone (FSH) that occur in midlife. FSH dilates the tiny blood vessels under the skin's surface. When blood rushes into the dilated capillaries, it feels like the room temperature is 98.6 degrees! Getting your heart rate and circulation up boosts your endorphin level, which makes you feel better overall while also helping your body adjust to temperature changes and cool down more efficiently. Even moderate exercise appears to help ease the frequency and severity of hot flashes.

The right mix of strength training and aerobic moves is important during menopause to avoid simply spiking body temperature and bringing on a hot flash. A walk, a yoga session, some repetitions with light weights or resistance bands, or a swim for some slow and steady laps can relax you, keep you fit and toned, and ease your hot flashes at the same time. Cooling down after you exercise also helps— slow your pace and do some gentle stretches to wind down your workout.

## Tone It Down

Stress worsens hot flashes—as any woman who has felt herself beginning to drip during a high-pressure meeting or in the middle of a (literally) heated conversation knows. When that prickly, hot feeling starts to come on in an intense situation, take slow, deep breaths to help keep your stress at bay. Excuse yourself for a restroom break, whether or not you need one, to diffuse the tension. Visualizing yourself somewhere cool—next to a waterfall; on a leafy, shaded forest path; or on a hushed, snow-covered mountain trail— can also help refocus your brain and relax you. Carry your anti-hot-flash tools with you too. Tuck a fan in your purse, along with a handkerchief or tissues in case you need them.

Keep a bottle of cool water within reach so you can sip it to cool down and calm down.

## Cool Nights

While these daytime strategies of the right foods, regular activity, and stress management will help to ease your night sweats, that's not all you can do. Here are a few more tips to help keep you dry and comfortable at night:

- Keep a comfortable ambient temperature in your room. A quiet fan on a low setting can help keep the room from getting stuffy while you sleep, which can trigger night sweats.

- Try a cooling pillow. Made with gel-filled beads or crystals, these pillows are designed to stay cool during the night. You can choose from the type you sleep on like a regular pillow or a smaller version that you keep next to your regular pillow and use only if you wake up feeling warm.

- Layer your bedding at night just as you layer your clothing during the day. Silk sheets, once a symbol of luxury only for the spoiled, make a cool foundation that can help keep moisture away from your skin. Top them with a couple of lightweight blankets rather than a heavy comforter.

- Sleep in a nightgown or pajamas made with moisture-absorbing fabric. Avoid cotton, polyester, and anything with even a slightly snug waistband.

- Remember that alcohol close to bedtime ups the likelihood that you'll wake up sweaty during the night.

- End your workout well before you go to sleep—at least three hours. Your sleep will be more restful, and you'll be less likely to break out in a night sweat.

## Other Unwanted Moisture

Lack of estrogen in menopause changes the tone and strength of pelvic muscles, which can lead to stress incontinence in some women. That's when pressure from a cough, laugh, or sneeze makes you expel a little urine. You may also have experienced urge incontinence during menopause—when the bladder squeezes or contracts when you're not prepared—nowhere near a restroom, as luck would usually have it, and you leak urine. These urinary problems can be uncomfortable and embarrassing, but today you'll learn how to gain better control of pesky leakage.

## Pump Up the Pelvic Floor

Urine leakage can be reduced by strengthening your pelvic floor with Kegel exercises. You may have done these exercises during pregnancy. Many women make the mistake of tightening the wrong muscles when they think they are doing Kegel exercises, and then give up in frustration because they don't see any improvement in their ability to hold in urine leaks.

Kegels aren't hard, but you do have to do them correctly to get the benefit. You simply pretend that you have to urinate and then hold it. When you do this, you are tightening the pelvic floor muscles. Be sure that you aren't inadvertently sucking in your stomach or squeezing your buttocks.

Do Kegels when your bladder is empty. Hold your pretend urine for ten seconds if you can, and repeat ten times. Don't worry if you can't hold for a count of ten at first—your muscles will get stronger as you repeat the exercises. Aim for three sets of Kegels a day. You can do them anywhere, anytime, lying down or sitting.

In addition to doing regular Kegel exercises, you can retrain your bladder to help you control the urge to urinate. To start, when you feel like you have to go, see if you can wait five minutes. Once you feel like you can hold your urine for five minutes fairly easily, increase the time to ten minutes. Keep increasing the time gradually until you're able to go for longer, comfortable periods of time without dashing to the restroom. This process helps your brain and bladder muscles learn how to hold your urine longer.

Another step in bladder retraining is to go to the bathroom on a schedule, say every hour. Gradually adjust the schedule to include longer times between scheduled trips to the bathroom. This kind of training program can help you gain more control over your body and can lessen the need for frequent, panicky searches for the nearest restroom. A bladder retraining program generally takes from three to twelve weeks to have a measurable effect. And if you're concerned about a possible accident while you're retraining your bladder, remember that you can always wear an ultrathin pad for peace of mind until you feel sure about your ability to go for longer periods of time without urinating.

If your weight is above the normal range for your height, this can contribute to urinary leakage problems too. Extra weight puts extra pressure on your pelvic muscles. You'll find that even modest amounts of exercise will build your muscles and help you improve your ability to hold the flow.

What you eat and drink affects urinary incontinence as well. Too much caffeine is a definite culprit. Some women find that limiting carbonated sodas and foods with citrus and tomatoes helps ease urine leaks. These foods and drinks may irritate the bladder and create a more frequent urge to go.

Just these simple changes will help you feel less damp and irritated as you go through your days and less prone to waking up in what feels like your own little pool at night. You won't have to do as much advance planning to scope out the nearest restroom at any destination, or on the way there. And you won't spend nearly as much time asking, "Is it hot in here?" or "Where's the ladies' room?" Getting a handle on your hot flashes, night sweats, and urine leaks means you get to spend more time feeling good and doing the activities you truly enjoy.

# MEDICATIONS

Much as we get out the health or car insurance policy only when someone falls ill or the fender gets crushed, many of us ignore the noise about hormone replacement therapy (HRT) until our symptoms demand that we do something. Then the information about HRT can seem overwhelming and alarming. Today is the day you can cut through some of the conflicting and confusing information about HRT so you have a clear, rational way to evaluate your options. And today you'll sort out other medication conundrums that you may have faced.

If you feel uncertain or alarmed about HRT, you're in good company. But here's an important point: HRT isn't so complicated that you have to throw up your hands and either say, "I'm not going to take hormones," or defer to whatever your doctor recommends. You can be an active participant in the decision.

For many women, fear and confusion about HRT began when results of the Women's Health Initiative started to emerge in 2002. This long-term health study, launched in 1991, involved more than 160,000 women ages fifty to seventy-nine and came with a whopping $625 million price tag. The study results confused and frightened many women and their physicians.

Let's look at some of the information the study yielded, and place it in a context you can use to think about your own HRT decision.

- In the Women's Health Initiative, women taking estrogen plus progestin, which is synthetic progesterone, had higher rates of heart attack, stroke, and breast cancer than the women who were taking placebo. That portion of the study was abruptly halted in 2002, and millions of women who had been taking HRT stopped.

- The estrogen-only portion of the study was stopped a year early in 2006, when results demonstrated a slightly increased risk of stroke.

- Updates on the study from further analysis seemed to cloud, not clarify, the picture. In postmenopausal women, estrogen did not elevate the risk of breast cancer, but it also did not help with the risk. A report focusing on timing of therapy showed that women who start HRT closer to menopause may have a reduced risk of heart disease.

- Further analysis examined long-term risk, demonstrating that estrogen plus synthetic progestin use for more than five years doubles annual risk of breast cancer.

- A follow-up study of women who participated in the estrogen-only part of the study revealed a lower incidence of breast cancers, and in younger estrogen-only users who were in their fifties, a lower incidence of heart attacks.

The dizzying information from the Women's Health Initiative has left many women believing their HRT choice is starkly divided: take the stuff and run very serious health risks, or take nothing and tough out the disruptive symptoms. Your decision about HRT is much more nuanced than that. And remember that the decision you make today about HRT, whether it's yea or nay, can change anytime you choose.

In the years Stephanie has spent helping women think through this decision, and guiding them in the conversations they have with their doctor, she reminds them of these key facts about HRT:

- This choice is individual to you, and what suits your best friend, sister, or colleague may not be best for you. Hormone therapy is not one size fits all.

- The hormone dosages and forms used by women who participated in the Women's Health Initiative are not your only option. The hormones used in this research were synthetic forms of estrogen, made from the urine of pregnant mares, and progestin, which is synthetic progesterone.

- A single, standardized dose of estrogen and progestin was used for all the women in the study. You have many other choices when it comes to dosage and strength of hormone medication.

- Bioidentical forms of estrogen, progesterone, and testosterone are available. These are prescription medications and are not to be confused with over-the-counter products. Bioidentical hormones differ from synthetic hormones in that they match the hormones your body produces, molecule for molecule. They are available as pills, skin creams, gels, and patches as well as vaginal rings, gels, creams, and tablets. No bioidentical hormones were used in the Women's Health Initiative study.

- No head-to-head studies compare synthetic hormones, like the ones used in the Women's Health Initiative, with prescription bioidentical hormones, for safety or efficacy. While enterprising doctors and celebrities hawk bioidentical hormones and claim they are better or more natural, we still need solid research that backs up these assertions.

- Given the choice, however, women who take prescription bioidentical hormones report symptom relief without the side effects often associated with synthetic hormones, such as headache, bloating, or worsening depression.

## Making Sense of Standardized Advice

We can count it as progress that HRT dosages are no longer standardized. But now it's the advice about HRT that has become standardized, and it's not all that helpful. In the aftermath of the Women's Health Initiative, women are vaguely counseled to "talk with their doctors about HRT" or "weigh their personal risks and benefits." This sounds like so much drivel. First, many physicians cannot or will not take the time necessary to sort through the myriad of HRT options and to develop an individualized plan. Second, no tools or science can make weighing your risks a precise process.

So where do you go from here in figuring out whether HRT is the best option to manage your symptoms? Here are three preliminary steps:

1. Think about the degree to which your symptoms interfere with your life—your relationships, your work, your overall way of being in the world. You don't have to live with disruptive symptoms. This is especially true if sleeplessness, severe hot flashes, depression, or lack of libido are taking a significant toll on your quality of life. The health of your bones should factor into your decision about HRT too. If a bone density test reveals that you are at significant risk of fracture, hormone replacement may improve your bone strength.

2. Make a list of self-help measures you have already tried to manage your symptoms. How well did these self-care tactics work? Are you willing to continue with any nutrition or exercise strategies? If you haven't tried changing your diet, increasing your level of activity, or reducing your stress, are you willing to try these steps first? It's important to keep in mind that HRT, if you choose to use it, is only one part of your health equation.

3. Make a short list of what you expect from HRT. Some examples might include: I want to sleep. I want to have more energy. I want relief from vaginal

dryness so I can enjoy sex again. I want to feel less depressed. I want my hot flashes to stop. This step is important, because although HRT has a place in managing symptoms for some women, it will not act as a cure-all. HRT also will not counteract a stress-filled life, a consistently unhealthy diet, or an entirely sedentary existence.

After you give the steps above some thought, you may decide that you want to take HRT either because your symptoms are not sufficiently alleviated with self-care or because right now you feel like you can't pay consistent enough attention to your eating patterns, exercise, or stress level. Some women, along with being nervous about their decision to try HRT, also feel embarrassed or guilty that they aren't tough enough or disciplined enough to cope with menopause without medication.

If that sounds like you, remember that medication exists to correct hormone imbalances for good reason. Don't judge yourself or your decision to use HRT, just as you wouldn't judge a woman with diabetes who uses insulin, which is also a hormone, to control the condition.

Now let's look at deciphering what to take, when, and for how long. If you opt for HRT, remember that bioidentical forms can help manage symptoms with fewer side effects than synthetic forms. These bioidentical hormones are commercially made prescription medications.

| Bioidentical Hormones | | | |
|---|---|---|---|
| Hormone | Brand Name | Form | Dosage |
| Estradiol (a type of estrogen) | Estrace | Pill<br>Vaginal cream 0.01% | Tablet = 0.5, 1, or 2 mg<br>Cream = Applicator delivers 2 to 4 g |
| | Alora, Climara, Esclim, Estraderm, Vivelle | Patch | Dosages range from 0.25 mg to 0.1 mg |
| | EstroGel 0.06% | Gel applied to skin | 0.75 mg |
| | Estring | Vaginal ring | 7.5 mcg per 24 hours; ring is worn for 90 days |
| | Divigel 0.1% | Gel applied to skin | 0.25, 0.5, or 1.0 g dosages |
| Estradiol acetate (a type of estrogen) | Femring | Vaginal ring | 0.05 mg/day or 0.10 mg/day, worn for 90 days |
| Estradiol hemihydrate | Vagifem | Vaginal tablet | 10 mcg or 25 mcg; tablet used once daily for two weeks, then twice weekly |
| Micronized progesterone USP (micronized means that the hormone is in very tiny particles to increase absorption) | Prometrium | Pill | 100 mg or 200 mg (contains peanut oil; cannot be used by women with peanut allergy) |
| | Crinone 4%<br>Crinone 8% | Vaginal gel | 4% = 45 mg<br>8% = 90 mg |

Bioidentical hormones can also be compounded individually by a compounding pharmacist. Individually compounded prescriptions have certain advantages: the dosages can be customized to deliver the smallest possible amount of medication. This can be a plus for women whose hormone levels are low but for whom the dosages of the commercial products are still too high.

The drawbacks of compounded prescription hormones include the fact that insurance plans rarely cover the cost. In addition, some physicians are unfamiliar with compounded preparations and mistakenly believe that you don't know what you are getting. They may not know what to prescribe.

A physician who is knowledgeable about bioidentical hormones understands that these are prescription medications, not unregulated over-the-counter products. They must be compounded by a registered pharmacist who uses prescription medications that meet US pharmacopeia standards.

## Lowest Dose, Shortest Duration

Whether you are going to choose commercially prepared or compounded hormone replacement, you'll want a regimen of the lowest dose and shortest duration possible. But what exactly does that look like? And how do you know what dose is right for you?

Your doctor may order a blood test to measure your estradiol (a type of estrogen), progesterone, and testosterone levels. Hormone levels can also be measured with saliva samples, but this option requires working with a physician who is familiar with this method as well as a credible lab to process the samples. The process involves collecting saliva samples by spitting into tubes at home, which you seal and ship to a laboratory. Some insurance plans do not cover this type of hormone testing, and some physicians are hesitant to order saliva hormone tests.

Your hormone test results give an indication of where you are on the hormone continuum and can help determine the degree to which low hormones are responsible for your symptoms. The hormone test is a useful part of the picture, but your subjective description of what you are experiencing carries equal weight. Sample blood test results may show something like this:

- Estradiol levels of less than 50 picograms/liter (pc/l) can occur in women who are still having periods but also have hot flashes, sleep disturbances, vaginal dryness, and other symptoms of low estrogen.

- Estradiol levels of less than 36 pc/l generally occur in women who are postmenopausal, whose periods have stopped altogether.

- Progesterone levels in menopausal women range between 0.03 and 0.3 nanograms/milliliter (ng/ml).

- A total testosterone level of less than 25 nanograms/deciliter (ng/dl) is generally considered deficient.

It's important to remember that these ranges are general. Two women with the same hormone levels may experience symptoms that differ significantly in severity. Both credible lab studies and your assessment of how you are feeling come into play in determining how to manage your menopause symptoms with medication.

Let's say you've told your doctor that your hot flashes are interrupting your sleep, and you have vaginal dryness, itching, and burning. Your hormone test indicates estradiol, progesterone, and testosterone levels below the normal range.

Your physician may prescribe a daily regimen that looks something like this: 0.25 or 0.5 mg of bioidentical estrogen and 50 to 100 mg of micronized progesterone. How long you take HRT depends on the symptoms you want to manage. Experts now agree that women should take HRT no longer than five years; many women find that a short course of HRT is enough to manage their symptoms until their bodies adjust and to get them over the hump, so to speak. If you choose to use HRT, think in terms of three-month increments. Assess how you feel, and work with your doctor to retest your hormone levels so your dosage can be adjusted as needed.

## Talk About Testosterone

A low dose of bioidentical testosterone—0.5 to 3 mg/day of a topical cream or gel—as part of a course of HRT can put the spark back into a stalled-out sexual drive for some women after menopause. This hormone also plays a role in increasing bone density and building lean muscle mass. Here's what's important to know about testosterone for women:

- Testosterone use in women is considered off-label. In other words, there is no product containing testosterone alone with FDA-approved labeling for women.

- The combination product that combines estrogen and testosterone that is FDA-approved for women, Estratest, contains synthetic estrogen, which tends to produce more side effects and should be avoided.

- Women with breast or uterine cancer cannot take testosterone.

- The commercial forms of bioidentical testosterone (Androderm and Androgel) are labeled as contraindicated for women.

- Women who use testosterone need to check in with their doctor every six to eight weeks to test their hormone levels and adjust the dosage as necessary.

- Bioidentical testosterone can be prescribed by your doctor and made by a compounding pharmacy.

## The Bottom Line

The decision you make about HRT isn't set in stone whether you decide yes or no. First, measure the difference made by healthier foods, more rest, less stress, and more fun activity. If those steps aren't providing adequate relief and you decide to try HRT, choose the bioidentical forms and see how you feel. Monitor your symptoms and evaluate whether they are easing up as much as you expected or would like. You know what's best for you. You've lived in your body your whole life, and you are the best judge of how you feel. Whether you decide to take HRT or not, the most important thing for you to remember is that you'll emerge on the other side of the menopausal transition with the same strength and resilience that carried you through all the other challenges in your life.

## What About Antidepressants?

The allure of antidepressants may seem even stronger to women in menopause than it has at any other point in their lives. A pill you can take seemingly indefinitely to dull the edges of depression may have a certain appeal, especially when you consider that the decision about antidepressants doesn't seem nearly as fraught with complex, confusing information as one about HRT. Many women simply don't want to adjust their lifestyle to include more activity or a healthier eating plan, yet they don't want to feel the way they do in menopause: flat, joyless, and irritable. What about getting through menopause with the help of an antidepressant?

Most antidepressants work by keeping the feel-good chemical serotonin in your brain longer than it would be otherwise. The name of the medication category, selective serotonin reuptake inhibitors, or SSRIs, describes that function. SSRIs have a place in the treatment of depression, and for many people, they are a lifesaver. And while feeling depressed is often on the top of the list of women's symptoms in menopause, in many instances these feelings do not result from clinical depression but from diminished or sporadic hormone production. Hormones serve as natural coping chemicals, and when they're in short supply during menopause, we can feel as if we're coming undone.

Current data from the Centers for Disease Control (CDC) states that 23 percent of women ages forty to fifty-nine take antidepressants, more than any other age or sex group. A large percentage of these women may actually be experiencing symptoms of perimenopausal or menopausal hormone disruption, not clinical depression. Many of them have no personal or family history of depression, yet they are now labeled as depressed. Our culture is such, and the nature of our health care system is such, that antidepressants are often represented as a quicker and easier fix than figuring out what's going on with estrogen, progesterone, and testosterone. It's understandable that a woman who feels mired in depression may say she doesn't have the energy or wherewithal to try some other steps first, like eating nourishing foods and going out for a walk three times a week.

Before you take the antidepressant route, it's important to know what you can and cannot expect from this type of medication. These medications take awhile to start working—between ten days and two weeks—there are no overnight results. Antidepressants can take the edge off what can seem like a black cloud of despair. But when taking antidepressants, many women experience a flat feeling. The profound lows of their previously depressed state may not seem so acute. Many women describe feeling stuck in neutral, with no highs, no joyful sparks, and no surges of excitement or happiness either. Antidepressants can also diminish sexual desire and response. Many menopausal women are looking for something to help them with low sex drive, not a medication that either brings this symptom on or worsens it.

Then there is weight gain associated with antidepressants. That's the part they don't talk about on the TV ads for antidepressants that show the woman gazing wistfully out the window (she isn't chunky) or in the slick magazine pages depicting a trim woman in workout clothes frolicking in a meadow with her Frisbee. Approximately one-fourth of people who take antidepressants gain ten pounds or more, usually if they have taken the antidepressant for more than six months. Scientists aren't sure whether these medications wield some kind of influence on metabolism that accounts for the weight gain or if emerging from a fog of depression helps people to feel more interested in food and eating again. But this is something to be aware of.

Many women start taking an antidepressant to manage feeling depressed but then become very unhappy about the extra weight, especially around the middle, that they have to deal with. It's important to understand that antidepressants cannot be stopped suddenly—the dosage must be tapered down gradually. This can take weeks or months, depending on the specific antidepressant they are taking, how long they've taken it, the dosage, and whether they have recurring symptoms when the dose is gradually reduced.

Frequently, women who take an antidepressant during what feels like a particularly bad patch find that once they stop taking the medication, their feelings of depression return. As a result, they are often told that they need to consider taking the medication indefinitely. In some cases, with women who truly have clinical depression that can't be managed otherwise, this may be appropriate. However, in many instances, the recurring depression stems from discontinuing antidepressants too abruptly. In fact, withdrawing from antidepressants too suddenly, without carefully tapering the dosage, can produce a host of unpleasant, flu-like symptoms, including body aches and fever. In addition, the withdrawal from antidepressants can produce an even flatter mood, which then convinces many women that they have to go back on the medication, and the cycle begins again.

## Other Medications for Hot Flashes

Antiseizure medications are sometimes prescribed to control severe hot flashes in women, defined as seven or more a day. This is considered an off-label use of these medications because the drugs are meant to treat epilepsy or severe pain that follows shingles, not hot flashes. A couple of small studies measuring the effectiveness of the antiseizure medication gabapentin in alleviating hot flashes showed that women taking the drug did have a significant drop in hot flashes. The drug can produce side effects including dizziness, sleepiness, and swelling. There are many other ways to tame hot flashes—you learned about them on Day 8—other than drugs meant to prevent convulsions.

# Thyroid Medication

The symptoms of menopause overlap with symptoms caused by low thyroid, or hypothyroidism: stubborn weight gain, diminished sex drive, trouble sleeping, a foggy feeling or difficulty concentrating, and hair loss or thinning hair.

But here is the tricky part: a single test of thyroid-stimulating hormone (TSH) often isn't enough to indicate whether you are deficient in thyroid hormones because this test can vary according to season, time of day, your activity level, and your overall health. Up to a third of people whose TSH test indicates a slightly elevated level will find that the level is normal when retested within a few months.

If you suspect that low thyroid is causing or compounding your menopause symptoms, talk with your doctor about whether testing your TSH, as well as your free T3 and free T4—the thyroid hormones themselves—is appropriate. Remember that thyroid issues can coexist with menopause, and it's not an either/or situation. A normal thyroid test may warrant retesting down the road if symptoms continue, and it's important not to overlook the possibility that thyroid function can be part of the picture if fatigue, hair loss, depression, and lack of sex drive are your most troubling symptoms. Many women find that boosting their nutrition and reducing their stress level help mitigate these symptoms, but women whose thyroid level is consistently below the normal range may need to supplement with this hormone.

## No Bones About It

Do I need to take medication to prevent bone loss? Many women ask that question, unsure about their risk. We've all seen the TV commercials featuring beautiful, mature stars with lithe bodies and thick manes of silver hair, touting the benefits of drugs to prevent osteoporosis.

When the first bisphosphonate was approved in 1995 to treat and prevent osteoporosis, it was often prescribed to women who had a bone density test with lower than normal results but who did not have osteoporosis. The thinking was that the bisphosphonate would prevent the progression of the disease, and women took the drug indefinitely.

That thinking has changed now. More recent data shows that osteoporosis develops very slowly, according to a study of five thousand women conducted by University of California, San Francisco researchers. This study, along with a CDC report showing that more than 70 percent of women older than sixty-five did not have osteoporosis, has prompted experts to revise the way they approach the issue of bone health for women in menopause. There was a time when it seemed as if women were constantly being warned that their bones were going to crumble. We know now that this isn't the case for most women.

Bisphosphonates do prevent fractures in people who already have osteoporosis, but they are no longer recommended to prevent the disease in people who do not have it. In addition, because bisphosphonates are associated with rare but serious side effects—bone loss in the jaw and fracture of the thighbone—they are now prescribed for no more than five years, mostly to older people who have osteoporosis, and no longer to younger, postmenopausal women.

The news is good: most women do not develop osteoporosis, and you don't necessarily need to reach into your medicine cabinet to avoid joining those who do.

## Over-the-Counter Medications and Supplements

Stephanie's recommendation to women on over-the-counter medications and supplements is pretty easy: save your money. Yes, soy milk stirred into your coffee or some crisp tofu in a stir-fry will be fine, but soy tablets have not proven to provide any relief from menopausal symptoms, according to the *Annals of Internal Medicine*. The same goes for flaxseed—delicious to eat and a good source of healthy fatty acids, but research data from the Mayo Clinic showed no difference in hot flashes between postmenopausal women who consumed flaxseed and those who took a placebo. You may also have heard or read that black cohosh, red clover, dong quai, evening primrose oil, ginseng, wild yam extract, chaste tree, hops, sage leaf, or kava kava can ease menopause symptoms, but there is still no strong evidence supporting any of these claims.

## Medication Mottos

- Try non-drug solutions first. Review what you have learned from this ten-day plan and trust in your ability to help yourself feel better. Give yourself the time you need to focus on your health. If, after four to six weeks, you find that your menopause symptoms still interfere significantly with your ability to function and enjoy life, let your doctor know you'd like to try bioidentical HRT as a next step.

- Choose bioidentical prescription forms. If you opt for HRT, tell your doctor that you prefer a bioidentical prescription form and that you want to start at the bottom of the dosage range. Keep notes on how your symptoms differ when you take the medication, and assess the degree of relief the medication provides. Be sure to write down how you are feeling in order to keep a complete and accurate record. This is easier and more thorough than relying on your memory.

- Set a date to stop HRT. Be sure your doctor understands that you want to wean off HRT as soon as possible. Plan to check in with your doctor every three months while you are taking hormone therapy. When you are ready, you and your doctor can develop a plan to reduce the dosage gradually, generally over a period of three months.

Many women find that a short course of bioidentical HRT offers a welcome period of symptom relief, allowing them to get some much-needed rest and restore their equilibrium. Women often find that after they discontinue HRT, their bodies have adjusted to this new phase in their lives and their symptoms are much more manageable, if they are present at all.

Just as women aren't ill when they're menstruating or pregnant, women in menopause do not have a condition that must always be medicated. Yet the symptoms of these hormonal events in women's lives sometimes do require medication. That's true of extremely severe morning sickness or brutal menstrual cramps that interfere with functioning as well. It may also be the case for you during menopause if sleeplessness, anxiety, depression, or other symptoms get in the way of truly living each day.

# MEDITATION

You've spent nine days discovering new strategies to improve your physical and emotional health—congratulations! By implementing even a few of these tips every day as you go forward from here, you'll look and feel newly energized, rest better, nourish yourself with delicious and colorful foods, build your heart and bones, recharge your energy, and put the spark back in your life overall. Each of these accomplishments is an important part of your health and well-being. It's equally crucial to tend to your spiritual health, which is what you are going to focus on today.

So often, we women focus on everyone else's needs, neglecting our own and being unfaithful, in a sense, to ourselves. Finding and connecting with your spiritual core is both intensely personal to your beliefs, needs, and outlook as well as deeply necessary for strength and replenishment. Find time every day to stop, detach yourself momentarily from the hectic pace of ticking things off of to-do lists, and take part in a relaxing or meditative activity.

Being meditative isn't confined to posing in specific positions or chanting a mantra, although a meditation practice can include these things. You may be surprised to learn that you have the power to change the flow of your brain waves with what is called nondirected meditation, which you can do anywhere, anytime. It's a practice you can easily learn, and you will find that this simple, yet very powerful discipline brings lasting benefit and change to your days well beyond the menopausal years.

Research demonstrates that simply stopping for a few minutes to let the mind go where it will without trying to monitor or direct any thoughts results in increased theta and alpha waves in the brain. These brain waves indicate a relaxed, wakeful state even though the brain is not at rest. At the same time, merely taking a few minutes to allow the mind to wander slows down the beta waves in the brain, which occur when the brain is working on tasks such as planning or organizing. This simple process of increasing theta and alpha waves and decreasing beta waves taps in to your power and can result in a sharper attention span, improved memory, greater relaxation, and reduced stress. With nondirected meditation, your mind remains open and aware, but you take a few minutes to shift from the customary churning thoughts to a more peaceful form of consciousness.

With phones ringing, work piling up, family and coworkers clamoring for attention, the computer screen blinking, and possibly even pets expectantly waiting for you to serve them, you might think that finding time for meditation will be impossible. Here are the three main things to remember about daily meditative time:

1. It doesn't have to take hours. You can try nondirected meditation for just three to five minutes at a time.

2. Quiet, meditative time is just as important to your health as good food, rest, and exercise.

3. You can create your own meditative moments, in the style and at the time that pleases and suits you.

Where and when you choose to take this time is up to you. No one else can provide this calming and grounding experience for you, so take the opportunity to identify the forms of meditation that work best for you. Here are some suggestions:

- Before you reach for your car keys to get ready to rush off, close your eyes, rest your palms in your lap, and let your thoughts go for a few minutes. Can't turn off the chatter in your mind? If a thought or worry threatens to intrude on your few moments of peace, picture yourself placing those thoughts into a box labeled Not Now. You can also do this when you arrive at your destination—after you turn off the engine but before you get out of the car.

- Your meditation doesn't have to be silent if you don't want it to. What music helps you connect with the part of your being that is joyful and creative? Your favorite Latin, classical, jazz, country, or rock sound can be a peaceful soundtrack to your meditation. Keep the volume fairly low while you let your mind relax and declutter.

- The connection to the heart's core has spiritual meaning for many women. You may decide to practice your meditation for a few moments each day with a prayer that expresses your gratitude, hope, inspiration, or forgiveness.

- Think about invigorating your meditative exercise with an activity you do with your hands and enjoy. This might be knitting, embroidering, planting or arranging flowers, kneading bread, weaving, beading jewelry, sculpting with clay, or collaging a scrapbook page or handmade card. The key is to approach these activities not as a task or with a pre-conceived idea of how they should turn out or how long it should take to do them, but just as something to do mindfully, calmly. Some women even find certain household chores meditative, such as ironing, sifting through a drawer to tidy it up, slicing vegetables or fruit, or grooming a pet. When done thoughtfully and quietly, and with time to let the mind wander where it will, almost anything can be part of a reflective time with meaning and purpose.

- Bring humor and playfulness to your meditative time by connecting with children. Stop by the children's room on your next visit to the public library, pause for a moment at the park playground, or look and listen the next time you are walking or driving by a schoolyard. Without babysitting or being responsible, you can observe the intensity and earnestness that children bring to playing. Sometimes just watching exuberance and joy can be infectious.

- On Day 7, we described walking as a means not only to keep your heart and bones strong but also as a way to practice a form of moving meditation. This can be your regular stroll in the neighborhood or park, but treat yourself to the occasional moving meditation in a place where the colors, light, and sounds around you please the eye and the spirit. Stroll through a museum, tour the landscaped grounds or gardens at a historical site, visit a restored mansion, or amble along a placid lakefront. As you walk, let your thoughts go and allow your senses to take in what you hear, see, and smell. This style of promenade is an entirely different variety of power walk, focused more on awakening your calming and soothing brain waves.

Women often say flat out, "I can't do this." Or they say that they can't shut off the noise in their minds or that this kind of quiet time makes them feel anxious or even sad. It may seem a bit scary at first, to take this absolute time for yourself, brief as it may be, to listen to the language of the spirit. Remember that there are no *shoulds* when it comes to experiencing a meditative time—simply making the decision to stop for a few minutes every day is healthy and restorative. If you find yourself wrestling with feelings of sorrow or nervousness during a more quiet time, practice taking some deep breaths. Observe what you are feeling without trying to judge the emotion or make it go away. Think of these moments as an opportunity to learn something about yourself each time you let your mind enter into this state of relaxed awareness. If you are the type of woman who keeps very busy, so much so that a few unscheduled moments become unsettling, you may want to take this as your cue that you need more, not less, of this kind of uninterrupted, tranquil interlude.

Meditative time recharges your commitment to your health and renews your focus on the spirit. As a daily habit, meditation allows a reflective, thoughtful, or even prayerful time—whichever is most comfortable and familiar to you—that subtly shifts you from rushing around to a more deliberate way of thinking about what you are doing and why. When you meditate, you replenish the well that allows you to flourish in the fullness of all your experiences, both the positive and the not so great.

Menopause marks a new phase of your life, in which your needs differ from earlier desires or requirements. Remember that your symptoms are not permanent, and know that life brings new freedom and energy when you emerge on the other side of this passage. The ten days that you have spent turning your attention toward your physical, emotional, and spiritual health can be just the beginning of a succession of days that unfold with vigor, enjoyment, and strength. You can smooth the transition into menopause and beyond by continuing to practice the steps you have learned in the last ten days. Yes, this is a ten-day self-care plan, but paying attention to your health and well-being isn't a short-term task. Being mindful of what you eat and how you relax, spending time with optimistic and fun people, going outside, making sure that your rest is a priority—all these ways of nurturing yourself carry individual weight, yet their cumulative power can serve you well into your next decade and more. The benefits of caring for yourself spill over into your alertness and memory, your enjoyment of intimacy, and your sheer joy and gratitude to be here. In carrying forward what you discovered about your health and about yourself in these ten days, you claim this time as one of creativity, purpose, and power.

# AFTERWORD

We can scarcely imagine a time when a woman needed her husband's permission to apply for a credit card, but that was true only a little more than fifty years ago. That's when many women who will reach menopause in the next few years were born. The requirement assumed that a woman had no income to pay her own bills or that she'd spend recklessly without sensible male oversight. The notion seems like an outlandish relic from another century, but it was part of this generation

With a no-less-determined, but perhaps quieter, approach, women reaching menopause today are bringing seismic changes to this experience, just as women before us revolutionized the way we earn and spend money, wear pants, give birth, and hold elected office. The physical changes that go along with menopause may have changed very little, but we are profoundly altering the way we think and talk about this transition in life. We now know that we have the choice to move through this stage grateful for our health, enjoying our relationships and our work, proud of what we've accomplished, and anticipating all we still intend to do and learn. We've replaced the fear or furtiveness about menopause with the aplomb, style, energy, and knowledge we need to thrive.

After more than thirty years of working with women at Full Circle Women's Health and meeting them all over the country at conferences, lectures, and club meetings, Stephanie continues to be impressed with women's willingness to articulate their health concerns and share very personal stories. These women are generous in revealing solutions that have worked for them in the interest of helping other women, and they are committed to smoothing the path for younger women who will follow. They have raised an eloquent, passionate, and authentic voice. This book reflects much of their accumulated wisdom, grace, humor, and confidence, which she is thankful to have witnessed and is delighted to pass along.

# Resources

Here is a list of information sources and products that may help you follow this ten-day self-care plan for menopause. This list isn't meant to be exhaustive—it's simple and easy to use. Similar items are likely available in your local stores, but these online options are for those of you who prefer to click rather than shop in person.

## Day 1: Mark Your Calendars

You may decide to keep a journal or notes about your feelings and experiences during the ten days.

### Bound Journals

Any book with blank pages will do, of course, but here are some sources for lovely handmade journals if you decide to treat yourself.

- Creative Paper Online, *www.handmade-paper.us*
- Ex Libris Anonymous, *www.bookjournals.com*
- Luna Bazaar, *www.lunabazaar.com/blank-handmade-journals.aspx*
- Rustico, *www.rusticoleather.com*

### Digital Journaling

These apps let you keep your journal on your smartphone or tablet, complete with scribbles and images.

- Draw Pad Pro, Available on iTunes
- Evernote, *www.evernote.com*
- Livescribe, *www.livescribe.com*
- Momento, *www.momentoapp.com*
- PhatPad, *www.phatware.com*
- Wonderful Days, *www.wonderfuldayapp.com*

# Day 2: Mood

Conducting research on your sleep habits and what they mean can be a great place to start improving your mood.

- The National Sleep Foundation, *www.sleepfoundation.org*

Also consider earplugs to help enhance your sleep and mood. The Hearos earplug has received high ratings for comfort and noise reduction.

- Earplug Superstore, *www.earplugstore.com*

Look for 100 percent mulberry silk with a momme weight of 19 or higher for the best quality in silk sheets. Here are a couple stores you can buy from online. Or shop your local bedding store or stalwart retailers like Sears and keep an eye out for sales.

- Feeling Pampered, *www.feelingpampered.com*
- True Mores Silk, *www.truemores.com*

Try a special anti-snoring pillow that keeps your head—or your partner's—gently tilted to the side to reduce snoring.

- The Sharper Image, *www.sharperimage.com*

Sources for full-length body pillows to support your back and to help keep you sleeping on your side include

- Bed Bath & Beyond, *www.bedbathandbeyond.com*
- Body Pillow Store, *www.bodypillowstore.net*
- MyComfortU, *www.mycomfortu.com*
- Tempur-Pedic, *www.tempurpedic.com*

Rely on soothing sounds to help you sleep and feel better. Try CDs or MP3s with natural sounds of the ocean, rainstorms, birdsong, and more.

- Nature Sounds, *www.nature-downloads.naturesounds.ca*
- Nature Sounds MP3, *www.naturesoundsmp3.net*
- Partners in Rhyme, *www.partnersinrhyme.com*
- Serenity Supply, *www.serenitysupply.com/catalog/ Nature-Sounds-4-1.html*

A relaxation app could do wonders for you.

- National Center for Telehealth and Technology, *www.t2health.org/apps/breathe2relax*

Volunteering to help others offers a way to lift your mood. The United Way site can help you identify volunteer opportunities in your community.

- The United Way, *www.unitedway.org*

# Day 3: Memory

Take a look at the Day 1 resources for journals and notebooks. A small notebook in your purse or on your nightstand gives you a handy way to jot down ideas so you don't have to worry about forgetting them.

Here is a sampling of online retailers where you can order delicious, memory-boosting chocolate:

- Bissingers, *www.bissingers.com*
- Cacao Atlanta Chocolate Co., *www.cacaoatlanta.com*
- L.A. Burdick, *www.burdickchocolate.com*
- Lake Champlain Chocolates, *www.lakechamplainchocolates.com*
- Li-Lac Chocolates, *www.li-lacchocolates.com*
- The Little Chocolate Company, *www.thelittlechocolatecompany.com*
- Rocky Mountain Chocolate Factory, *www.rockymountainchocolatefactory.com*
- V Chocolates, *www.vchocolates.com*
- Valerie Confections, *www.valerieconfections.com*

If you'd rather have your chocolate in pill form, cocoa supplements are available from these sources:

- CocoaVia, *www.cocoavia.com*
- Reserveage Organics, *cocoawell.org*

If you prefer your chocolate in savory rather than sweet form, Zingerman's has three types of mole sauces.

- Zingerman's, *www.zingermans.com*

# Day 4: Mirror

Donate the clothes you are retiring to organizations that need them.

- Dress for Success, *www.dressforsuccess.org*
- Goodwill Industries International, *www.goodwill .org*
- The Salvation Army, *www.salvationarmyusa.org*
- The Women's Alliance, *www.thewomensalliance.org*
- Your community theater or the drama department of your local high school

Your surplus of shoes can go to those in need.

- Soles 4 Souls, *www.soles4souls.org*

You could also decide to sell your clothing, shoes, and accessories through auction sites.

- Dresm, *www.dresm.com*
- eBay, *www.ebay.com*
- If the Shoe Doesn't Fit, *www.iftheshoedoesntfit.com*

To create your own home spa experience, choose a body scrub, bath salts, soap, or bath foam with a scent and texture you love. Whether you favor a dessert-like crème brûlée bath, a tingly ginger, or a restful rosemary, here are a few sources for your home spa necessities:

- Laura Mercier, *www.lauramercier.com*
- Level Naturals, *www.levelnaturals.com*
- San Francisco Bath Salt Company, *www.sfbsc.com*
- Two Little Blackbirds, *www.twolittleblackbirds.com*

Include a spritz of olive oil on dry skin.

- Misto Olive Oil Sprayer,
  *www.mistooliveoilsprayer.com*

Wrap up in a big, comfy bath sheet or treat yourself to a spa robe.

- Plush Necessities, *www.plushnecessities.com*
- Robeworks, *www.robeworks.com*
- Telegraph Hill Robes, *www.telegraphhill.com*

Light a candle with your favorite fragrance, or refresh your senses with a new aroma.

- Candle Delirium, *www.candledelirium.com*

# Day 5: Mojo

This is one reliable site for sex-enhancing toys:

- We-Vibe, *www.we-vibe.com*

Lubricant options include

- Astroglide, *www.astroglide.com*
- Firefly Organics, *www.fireflyorganics.com*
- Slippery Stuff, *www.slipperystufflubes.com*
- Vagisil, *www.vagisil.com*
- Wet Naturals, *www.wetnaturals.com*

# Day 6: Munchies

Many women have more cookbooks than they know what to do with. But sometimes a new one can be just the thing to help inspire you to try some different, healthy dishes. We list just a few here for their healthy recipes, beautiful writing, humor, and lovely photography.

- *The Art of Simple Food* by Alice Waters
- *The Greens Cookbook* by Deborah Madison
- *Heirloom Beans* by Steven Sando and Vanessa Barrington
- *Home Cooking: A Writer in the Kitchen* by Laurie Colwin
- *Stir-Frying to the Sky's Edge* by Grace Young

Carry your lunch and snacks in style with a tote that looks more like a purse.

- Built NY, *www.builtny.com/lunch-bags-totes-cat.html*
- Cool Tote, Inc., *www.coollunchbags.com/servlet/the-Purse-Style-Lunch-Bags/Categories*

A new reusable water bottle can help remind you to stay hydrated.

- Base Brands, *www.reduceeveryday.com*
- Camelbak Products, *www.camelbak.com*
- Nalgene, *www.nalgene.com*

# Day 7: Muscle and Bone

Find a walking trail in your area.

- TrailLink, *www.traillink.com*
- Trails, *www.trails.com*

You could even try to find walking club in your community.

- American Heart Association, *www.mywalkingclub.org/find-a-club*

Your local hospital or medical center, or your health plan, may also sponsor a walking group.

Check with your local parks and recreation department and community college for exercise classes and opportunities— these are often reasonably priced and offer a way to meet new people too.

Look fashionable while you keep fit by wearing something that makes you look as good as you feel.

- Athleta, *www.athleta.gap.com*
- Glamour Fitness, *www.glamour-fitness.com*
- Impact Fitness, *www.impactfitnesswear.com*
- Lululemon, *www.lululemon.com*

Find a flattering hat, too, to keep the sun off your head and face while you enjoy the outdoors in warm weather.

- Coolibar, *www.coolibar.com/womensunprotectiveclothing.html*
- Sunday Afternoons, *www.sundayafternoons.com*

Have a yoga session anytime without schlepping a yoga mat around. Yoga-Paws for your hands and feet let you do your routine anywhere.

- Yoga-Paws, *www.yogapaws.com*

Choose a flattering, comfortable swimsuit for any water exercise you decide to do.

- Lands' End, *www.landsend.com*
- Swimsuits for All, *www.swimsuitsforall.com*
- Venus Fashion, *www.venus.com*

Cultivate your garden as exercise. Here are some sources of heirloom and specimen plants and seeds, for variety and fun.

- Annie's Heirloom Seeds,
  *www.anniesheirloomseeds.com*
- Baker Creek Heirloom Seeds, *www.rareseeds.com*
- Granny's Heirloom Seeds,
  *www.grannysheirloomseeds.com*
- Rancho Gordo, *www.ranchogordo.com*
- Select Seeds, *www.selectseeds.com*
- Wild Boar Farms, *www.wildboarfarms.com*

# Day 8: Moisture

Moisture-wicking bedding and nightwear can help manage hot flashes and night sweats.

- Sleep Dry, Stay Cool, *www.sleepdrystaycool.com*

Resting your head on a cooling pillow can also help ease sweaty nights.

- Cooling Pillows, *www.coolingpillows.com*
- Polar Pillow, *www.polar-pillow.com*

A quiet fan can help keep you cool too.

- The Honeywell Quiet Set 8-Speed Tower fan is available at Target *(www.target.com)*.
- The Holmes HASF-1515 fan is available at Sears *(www.sears.com)*.

Thin pads can provide protection and peace of mind while you're strengthening your bladder muscle to control urine leaks.

- *www.poise.com*

## Day 9: Medication

Your doctor may order blood tests to measure your hormone levels. Saliva hormone testing can give you and your doctor additional information, but it's very important to use a credible laboratory.

- Aeron Life Cycles Clinical Laboratory, *www.aeron.com*

## Day 10: Meditation

You may want to write about your experience of meditation in a journal (see Day 1 resources).

Some women find guided meditation CDs helpful to get started with meditation. Other women prefer the short, nondirected style of meditation described in Chapter 10 and use guided meditation CDs occasionally for a deeper practice. Here are just a few of the more popular guided meditation CDs. You'll find many on Amazon or iTunes, where you can listen to samples and choose the style that suits you best.

- The Calming Collection: Goodbye Worries, Roberta Shapiro, *www.helpwithworry.com*

- Journey into Meditation, Lisa Guyman, *www.lisaguyman.com*
- Natural Awareness: Guided Meditations and Teachings for Welcoming All Experience, Pema Chödrön, *www.pemachodronfoundation.org/buy-cds-dvds/*
- Inner Journeys to Tranquility, Dr. Arlene Alexander, *www.sequoiarecords.com*

# ABOUT THE AUTHORS

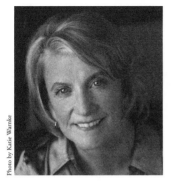

**STEPHANIE BENDER** was among the very first to voice the truth that the influence of women's hormones was not all in their heads, long before terms like *PMS* or *postpartum depression* were part of the national lexicon. Founder of Full Circle Women's Health in Colorado, she has significantly contributed to a much larger understanding of women's health through her books, lectures, and television appearances. This is her fifth book.

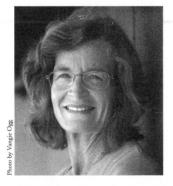

**TREACY COLBERT** is a medical writer. She is coauthor of *Before It's Too Late: What Parents Need to Know about Teen Pregnancy and STD Prevention* and *The Power of Perimenopause: A Woman's Guide to Physical and Emotional Health During the Transition Decade.* A graduate of Indiana University and the University of Wisconsin, she lives in Long Beach, California, with her husband and son.

# TO OUR READERS

Conari Press, an imprint of Red Wheel/Weiser, publishes books on topics ranging from spirituality, personal growth, and relationships to women's issues, parenting, and social issues. Our mission is to publish quality books that will make a difference in people's lives—how we feel about ourselves and how we relate to one another. We value integrity, compassion, and receptivity, both in the books we publish and in the way we do business.

Our readers are our most important resource, and we appreciate your input, suggestions, and ideas about what you would like to see published.

Visit our website at *www.redwheelweiser.com* to learn about our upcoming books and free downloads, and be sure to go to *www.redwheelweiser.com/newsletter* to sign up for newsletters and exclusive offers.

You can also contact us at *info@redwheelweiser.com*.

Conari Press
an imprint of Red Wheel/Weiser, LLC
665 Third Street, Suite 400
San Francisco, CA 94107